SOLUTIONS *for* SUCCESS

A Training Manual for Working with Older People Who Are Visually Impaired

SOLUTIONS *for* SUCCESS

A Training Manual for Working with Older People Who Are Visually Impaired

ALBERTA L. ORR

PRISCILLA ROGERS

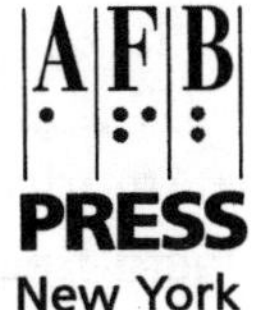

New York

Printed in the United States of America.

This publication was made possible by a generous grant from The Merck Company Foundation.

Library of Congress Cataloging-in-Publication Data

Orr, Alberta L., 1950–

Solutions for success : a training manual for working with older people who are visually impaired / Alberta L. Orr, Priscilla Rogers.

p. cm.

Includes index.

ISBN 0-89128-859-7

1. Aged people with visual disabilities—Rehabilitation. 2. Aged people with visual disabilities—Care. I. Rogers, Priscilla. II. Title.

RE48.2.A5 O735 2002

618.97'77—dc21

2002034518

The American Foundation for the Blind—the organization to which Helen Keller devoted more than 40 years of her life—is a national nonprofit whose mission is to eliminate the inequities faced by the 10 million Americans who are blind or visually impaired.

It is the policy of the American Foundation for the Blind to use in the first printing of its books acid-free paper that meets the ANSI Z39.48 Standard. The infinity symbol that appears above indicates that the paper in this printing meets that standard.

CONTENTS

APPENDIXES

PREFACE

As more and more people in the United States and other countries are living longer, more of them are also encountering physical conditions and health problems associated with aging, including some degree of vision loss. Already, some 15 percent of people over the age of 65 have a loss of vision severe enough to interfere with everyday activities. Individuals who work with older people every day, however, often feel that they lack the knowledge and skills to help their clients who have visual impairments.

The staff of the National Aging Program of the American Foundation for the Blind set out to address that gap through the development of this curriculum and its companion video, *Solutions for Everyday Living for Older Individuals with Visual Impairments*. This training manual contains basic information about vision and age-related vision loss, as well as instruction in how people with visual impairments can carry out their everyday activities independently and safely. It can enable staff members of assisted living and other facilities to help older people who are visually impaired retain or regain their ability to function at their individual maximum level.

The content of this curriculum is useful for a variety of audiences because most of the skill areas covered are also appropriate for a broad array of hands-on professionals and paraprofessionals. It was initially designed for staff working in assisted living settings because that is one of the fastest growing living arrangements for older people in the country. It is also appropriate for staff members at any facility where older people live, however, such as nursing homes and continuing care retirement communities, as well as in such community-based settings as home health care and senior centers. The curriculum is intended to be taught by a staff member who is responsible for carrying out in-service training within the organization, but the format is designed to be user friendly so that staff members can study the key points and use the manual for reference after the training.

Through the generous support of The Merck Company Foundation, the authors developed and piloted the curriculum with staff in assisted living and continuing care retirement communities around the country. The curriculum was piloted in seven facilities:

Anchin Pavilion, Sarasota, FL
Laurelwood at the Highlands, Pittsford, NY
Mark Hill Village, Sevierville, TN
Masonic Home, St. Petersburg, FL
Medford Leas, Medford, NJ
Montebello on Academy, Albuquerque, NM
Shannondale Health Care, Knoxville, TN

The authors are grateful to the staff and residents of these facilities for making this publication possible, with special thanks to Laurelwood at the Highlands, the site of the companion video.

INTRODUCTION

The goal of this training manual is to help you recognize vision loss in older residents. Once you have learned about vision loss, the curriculum will provide you with the information you need to help individuals with vision loss function as independently as possible within your facility.

Why Is Learning about Vision Loss So Important?

People are living longer than ever before, and vision loss is closely associated with aging. Over 5 million individuals age 65 and older and 6.5 million age 55 and older in this country experience vision loss. This number of older persons with vision loss will continue to grow dramatically as middle-aged persons enter old age.

Age-related vision loss is caused by eye conditions such as

- macular degeneration
- glaucoma
- diabetic retinopathy
- complicated cataracts

These conditions are discussed in more detail in Lesson 3.

As a result of visual impairment, many older individuals have problems with carrying out normal activities. They may have problems with such activities as

- getting around
- using a telephone
- corresponding
- reading
- shopping
- preparing meals

They are also more likely to experience falls resulting in a broken hip.

Understanding Residents Who Are Experiencing Vision Loss

An older person who has recently lost vision may have experienced or may be currently experiencing a variety of other losses. It is important for you to know and understand how vision loss can affect older people and how they may be feeling.

FEELINGS OF OLDER PEOPLE WITH VISION LOSS

- They may feel the need to depend on someone else for everything.
- They may feel out of control.
- They may be afraid or unable to move about safely indoors or outdoors.
- They may have intense feelings about becoming unable to drive a car.
- They may feel cut off from the world.
- They may feel they have lost their privacy when someone has to read their personal mail or help in paying bills.
- They may think people are staring at them when they are using a cane, being guided by another person, or using a magnifier in a public place.
- They may feel cut off when in a group or with family members if they are unable to see gestures and facial expressions.
- Along with a loss of independence, they may experience feelings of inadequacy, low self-confidence, low self-esteem, and low self-worth.
- They may feel useless and unable to help others in some meaningful way.
- They may think they have to give up recreational and leisure activities.
- They may experience loss of income and incur increased costs as a result of vision loss.

Many residents may already be upset and depressed because they have recently lost their homes or a spouse or a good friend. Vision loss may increase depression, and it is especially hard for individuals who have always valued their independence. Many people also feel afraid because of their vision loss. In fact, visual impairment is one of the most feared disabilities in this country. But, as you will learn in this training guide, by learning adapted ways to carry out routine activities, residents may be able to adjust to their different life circumstances.

How Can I Help Residents with Visual Impairments?

You can help residents to regain independence, self-confidence, and self-esteem.

Many residents who experience a visual impairment will be able to do most things for themselves if they receive some instruction, help, and encouragement from you. It is also important to remember that if residents have difficulty with your instructions or are unresponsive to your suggestions or assistance, it may be that they have other health or physical concerns that limit their interest and abilities.

One of the most important things you can do to help residents who are visually impaired is to assist them in solving problems that occur as a result of vision loss. As a caregiver, you can learn how to help residents by applying simple solutions to such problems. There are seven key solutions that are easy to remember and that will be explained in detail in this manual.

KEY SOLUTIONS TO PROBLEMS CAUSED BY VISION LOSS

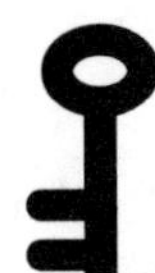

- use of large print
- use of devices with speech output
- use of contrast
- use of labeling techniques
- use of organizational techniques and systems
- use of tactile indicators and devices that make use of the resident's sense of touch
- use of environmental cues and techniques that make it safer and easier to get around in the facility

How This Guide Can Help You

This guide is intended to give you the information and techniques you need to know to help residents with visual impairments continue to live as independently and safely as possible. However, some of their needs require additional professional assistance. Appendix B of this manual provides sources for additional information and referrals for additional services. Catalogs of independent living aids are listed and can be ordered for use in some of the learning exercises included in this manual.

This training manual is divided into 20 lessons, each dealing with a different aspect of visual impairment and daily living. The first five lessons make up the core of the curriculum and should always be taught when this manual is utilized. To enable you to understand more about vision loss and how it affects older residents, two of the lessons include information about vision and eye diseases and conditions that affect older persons.

The other 15 lessons address ways to help residents carry out specific everyday tasks. You will want to review these lessons to determine which are critical to cover; this will depend on the residents in your facility and their particular type of vision loss and needs.

The manual begins with a pretest of your knowledge of visual impairment. You also will have a chance to take a posttest to determine how much information you have learned.

Each lesson has the following sections:

- goals—the overall aim of the lesson
- objective(s)—specific knowledge or ability to be gained from the lesson
- TEACH principles—important principles for working with older people who are visually impaired (as explained in Lesson 1)
- lesson content—the substance of the lesson; the core information to be learned
- key points—summary of the lesson content
- learning activities—activities for practicing what has been learned
- self-check—test of knowledge learned in the lesson

The text is accompanied by photographs and sketches that illustrate how to help residents learn to carry out particular activities.

A video entitled *Solutions for Everyday Living for Older People with Visual Impairments* is also available from AFB Press of the American Foundation for the Blind (see Appendix B) and can be used as a companion to this guide. It is recommended that you watch the video first as an overview before going through this written guide.

Note: Because this manual is written specifically about residents who have vision loss, the word *resident* always refers to a person who is visually impaired. Any exceptions will be noted in the text.

Now, please take a moment to complete the following pretest before starting the lessons. You will have the opportunity to take this same test at the end of the training to assess what you have learned.

Pretest on Age-Related Vision Loss

Indicate whether each statement is true (T) or false (F) in the space provided. The answers to the test can be found in Appendix A.

______ 1. Normal changes in the eye as people grow older include need for more light, presbyopia, and myopia.

______ 2. There are two types of visual field loss resulting from various eye conditions—central vision loss and side vision loss.

______ 3. The major eye diseases associated with aging are cataracts, macular degeneration, glaucoma, and diabetic retinopathy.

______ 4. Vision loss can be caused by stroke.

______ 5. Evaluating a resident's environment for glare, lighting, and contrast is a key strategy to help the older resident function more independently.

______ 6. Sighted guide is a technique used to teach guide dogs to guide individuals who are blind.

______ 7. Most people who experience age-related vision loss become totally blind.

______ 8. A resident who is experiencing sudden hazy or blurred vision, double vision, or recurring pain in or around the eyes should be checked as soon as possible by an eye care specialist.

______ 9. Loss of side vision can make tasks such as reading difficult for a resident.

______10. Writing is an activity that an older person with age-related vision loss has to give up.

PART 1 CORE LESSONS

LESSON 1 Key Principles of Working with Older Residents Who Are Visually Impaired

GOAL

To understand basic principles to keep in mind when working with older residents with visual impairments.

OBJECTIVE

At the end of the lesson, you will be able to discuss solutions to help older residents who are visually impaired function more independently.

TEACH Principles

When working with older persons with visual impairments, the overall goal is to help them to function as independently as possible. There are five important principles to remember that will assist residents in becoming independent. These are called the TEACH Principles.

THE TEACH PRINCIPLES

T stands for **Talking.** Talk to the resident. Tell him or her who you are and what you are doing. Explain things in very simple terms. Do not walk away from the resident without saying that you are leaving.

E stands for **Encouragement.** Encourage the resident to do things for him- or herself. Remind the resident of any devices and appliances he or she may have that will help him or her use vision, such as a cane, magnifier, or writing guide.

A stands for **Assess.** Be aware of the type of visual impairment the resident has and assess how that visual impairment affects the ability to carry out everyday tasks. You will need to reassess if the situation changes—if, for example, a resident experiences additional vision loss. You will also need to be able to assess the environment—including the resident's room and the common spaces in the facility—to determine if any changes can be made to help the resident see more clearly.

C stands for "**Can do.**" Remember, the resident can still do most daily living tasks and other personal tasks if shown ways to accomplish them. An older person with visual impairment may need your assistance at first, however, to relearn how to accomplish a task in a different way that he or she may have done all his or her life.

H stands for **Helping** the resident to regain control of his or her life. This may mean helping to organize personal items in the resident's room or apartment in a way that makes sense to the resident and makes items easy to find, or teaching the resident a way to find his or her own way to the dining room.

Remember the TEACH principles every time you come in contact with an older resident who is visually impaired. These principles will appear in all the lessons that involve helping residents learn new skills, lessons 5 through 20.

Solutions for Living with Visual Impairment

Learning about solutions that can be used to address and solve problems related to vision loss will help you as you begin to work with older residents who are visually impaired, helping them with daily activities. The seven key solutions are as follows:

SEVEN KEY SOLUTIONS

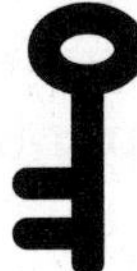

- use of large print
- use of devices with speech output
- use of contrast
- use of labeling techniques
- use of organizational techniques and systems
- use of tactile indicators and devices that make use of the resident's sense of touch
- use of environmental cues and techniques that make it safer and easier to get around in the facility

The following are brief overviews of each of these solutions.

LARGE PRINT

Older individuals who experience age-related vision loss may not be able to read regular print. They may need to have reading material in large print—

> print of this size, which is a type size of 18 points, or larger

—to read menus, activity schedules, signs, newspapers, or books.

DEVICES WITH SPEECH OUTPUT

Today's technology has made "talking" devices—tools or appliances that simulate speech—easily available to the public. Some examples are talking clocks and watches, talking weight scales, talking thermometers, and talking glucometers.

CONTRAST

Use of contrast means placing objects together that have a different appearance so that they stand out against each other and become more visible. Using colors that contrast to make print more legible is one example of using contrast effectively. White print on black paper or black print on beige or pale-yellow paper generally provides good color contrast for older persons with age-related vision loss (depending on the type of vision loss they have). White paper sometimes causes glare, reflecting light into the eye, even when the paper is not glossy. (See Lesson 2 for more information about glare.)

Similarly, improving the contrast between objects in the environment (putting dark towels in a white bathroom, for example) is one of the simplest and most effective ways to make the environment safer for residents.

LABELING TECHNIQUES

Different kinds of special labels can be used to help persons who are visually impaired recognize the correct medication, know what is in a can of food, or put on clothes whose colors match. Some methods of labeling that visually impaired residents can use are large-print and tactile indicators (which are explained later in the section on tactile indicators and devices).

ORGANIZATIONAL TECHNIQUES

Organizational techniques refer to having a system for storing and finding one's possessions. It is a key principle for helping older persons with visual impairments function well in their environment. Having a system that an individual develops and uses helps him or her to remain independent and in control of the environment. The old saying "everything in its place and a place for everything" is an important guideline.

TACTILE INDICATORS AND DEVICES

Tactile indicators or markers are objects that can be used for labeling by making use of the sense of touch, as discussed previously. A good example is a raised dot made out of plastic with a peel-and-stick backing that can be placed on stoves, microwaves, and thermostats to help a resident feel the correct setting. Another example is a braille clothing tag that indicates color with one or two braille letters.

One product to use for tactile markings is called Hi-Marks. It is a bright-orange liquid substance that hardens as it dries, making a raised bump that can be felt. (Hi-Marks and other marking products are available from the catalogs listed in Appendix B.)

ENVIRONMENTAL CUES AND TECHNIQUES

Making use of cues in the environment to give residents information about the surroundings will make it easier and safer for residents to walk around in the living environment. Using good lighting and good color contrast are two such techniques. A change in the texture of the floor covering can be used to indicate certain areas in the environment such as exits, common areas, and dangerous slopes. Sound is also a good environmental cue.

These seven key solutions will be explained in detail in the lessons throughout this curriculum, including when and how to use them to help older residents with visual impairments.

Congratulations! You have finished Lesson 1. Now go on to the Key Points to review what you have learned in this lesson. You will find these at the end of each lesson.

KEY POINTS IN LESSON 1

Key Principles of Working with Older Residents Who Are Visually Impaired

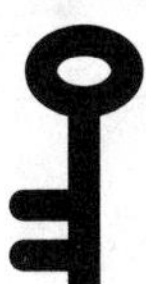

There are seven key solutions to helping an older person with visual impairment cope with vision loss:

- use of large print
- use of devices with speech output
- use of contrast
- use of labeling techniques
- use of organizational techniques and systems
- use of tactile indicators that make use of the resident's sense of touch
- use of environmental cues and techniques that make it safer and easier to get around in the facility

LEARNING ACTIVITIES

- Explain three of the key solutions for individuals with low vision.
- Brainstorm situations in which each solution can be used effectively.

☑ SELF-CHECK

You will find a self-check section at the end of each lesson to allow you to find out what you have learned and help you identify sections you may need to review before moving on to the next lesson.

Indicate whether each statement is true (T) or false (F) in the space provided. Check Appendix A for the answers. Then go back and review any statements you may have missed.

______ 1. Using labeling techniques is one way a resident can determine what clothing she is selecting to wear.

______ 2. White print on a dark background is an example of using contrast.

______ 3. Talking to the resident and encouraging the resident to try new techniques are two important TEACH principles.

LESSON 2

Normal Changes in the Aging Eye

GOAL

To understand the normal changes that occur in the eye as people age so that they can be distinguished from eye conditions or diseases that result in vision loss.

OBJECTIVE

At the end of the lesson you will be able to discuss normal age-related changes in the eye and how these changes can affect an individual's independence and ability to perform activities of daily living.

Normal Changes in the Aging Eye

Many changes occur in the eye as a result of growing older. These are normal results of the process of aging. Following are some of the most common changes:

- presbyopia
- reduced visual acuity
- increased need for light
- difficulty adapting to light and dark
- difficulty with glare
- reduced contrast sensitivity
- reduced ability to see colors
- reduced ability to see depth
- floaters
- dry eyes

Each of these changes will be explained in the sections that follow.

PRESBYOPIA

Presbyopia refers to a loss of the eye's ability to focus at close range. This is referred to as loss of *accommodation*. For example, an individual may begin to need to hold his or her reading material at arm's length to bring the print into focus. Presbyopia usually begins in midlife at approximately age 40.

SOLUTIONS FOR PRESBYOPIA

Presbyopia is correctable with eyeglasses: either reading glasses or eyeglasses that contain more than one prescription, such as bifocals, trifocals, and continuous-range eyeglasses.

REDUCED VISUAL ACUITY

Visual acuity is the ability to see objects clearly. A normal visual acuity for an older person is 20/40 with the best possible corrective lenses. By contrast, good vision for the average younger person is 20/20.

An individual who has a visual acuity of 20/40 sees at 20 feet what the person with 20/20 vision sees at 40 feet. A person with reduced visual acuity will have a hard time reading or distinguishing objects at a distance.

SOLUTIONS FOR REDUCED VISUAL ACUITY

Residents who are havng trouble seeing clearly may need an eye examination to determine whether eyeglasses will improve their visual acuity.

INCREASED NEED FOR LIGHT

The amount of light reaching the back of the eye commonly decreases with age. In the aging eye, a smaller pupil and increased haziness of the older lens of the eye causes the amount of light reaching the back of the eye to decrease dramatically, resulting in a need for increased lighting to see things clearly.

The average older person requires four times more light than a younger person. Older persons in their 80s require 10 times more light than people in their 20s.

SOLUTIONS FOR INCREASED NEED FOR LIGHT

Providing increased illumination from a light source that does not produce glare is the best solution to the need for more light. There are a number of lighting products on the market that can be helpful; they will be discussed in Lesson 4.

DIFFICULTY ADAPTING TO LIGHT AND DARK

Older adults often have difficulty adapting to changes in the level of light. In particular, the ability to adjust to darkness decreases with age. A good example is difficulty adjusting to the darkness of a movie theater after going in from the sunlight.

Adjusting from light to dark is generally harder than adjusting from dark to light. Adapting to a dark room can take an older person as long as 20 minutes. When an older person leaves a dim building lobby and walks outdoors into bright sunlight, adapting to the change in light usually occurs more quickly—in about 7 to 8 minutes.

SOLUTIONS TO ADAPTING TO LIGHT AND DARK

The best solution to problems with adapting to changes in light levels is to stay in one place or sit down after entering a dimly lit space until the eyes adjust to darkness.

DIFFICULTY WITH GLARE

Glare results when bright light enters the eye. The light may either shine directly on or be reflected into the eye. Glare can be caused by bright light reflecting from shiny surfaces such as a glass tabletop, highly polished floors, metal objects, or mirrors.

The ability to recover from bright lights and glare starts to decrease at around age 50. When there is glare in the environment, older people generally have difficulty distinguishing objects from their background. Too much glare can reduce vision.

Additional sources of glare include

- highly polished tile, linoleum, or wooden floors
- shiny desks or tabletops, and computer monitors
- reflective wall coverings, including glossy paint
- chrome fixtures, mirrors, and glossy tile in bathrooms
- uncovered lightbulbs in lamps and ceiling fixtures
- windows without curtains or shades in rooms, hallways, and dining areas

SOLUTIONS TO GLARE

You can help the resident function more independently by reducing sources of glare. For example, you may observe that a resident has stopped watching television. The resident may no longer be able to see the TV picture because the set is positioned in such a way that sun is shining directly on the screen. Moving the TV so that light is no longer shining on it may solve the problem for the resident.

Blinds are an effective window covering that can be adjusted to reduce glare. For bright, glary outdoor situations, sunglasses and a hat with a broad brim are useful.

REDUCED CONTRAST SENSITIVITY

Contrast sensitivity refers to the ability to detect differences between light and dark areas. Increasing the contrast between an object and its background generally makes the object more visible.

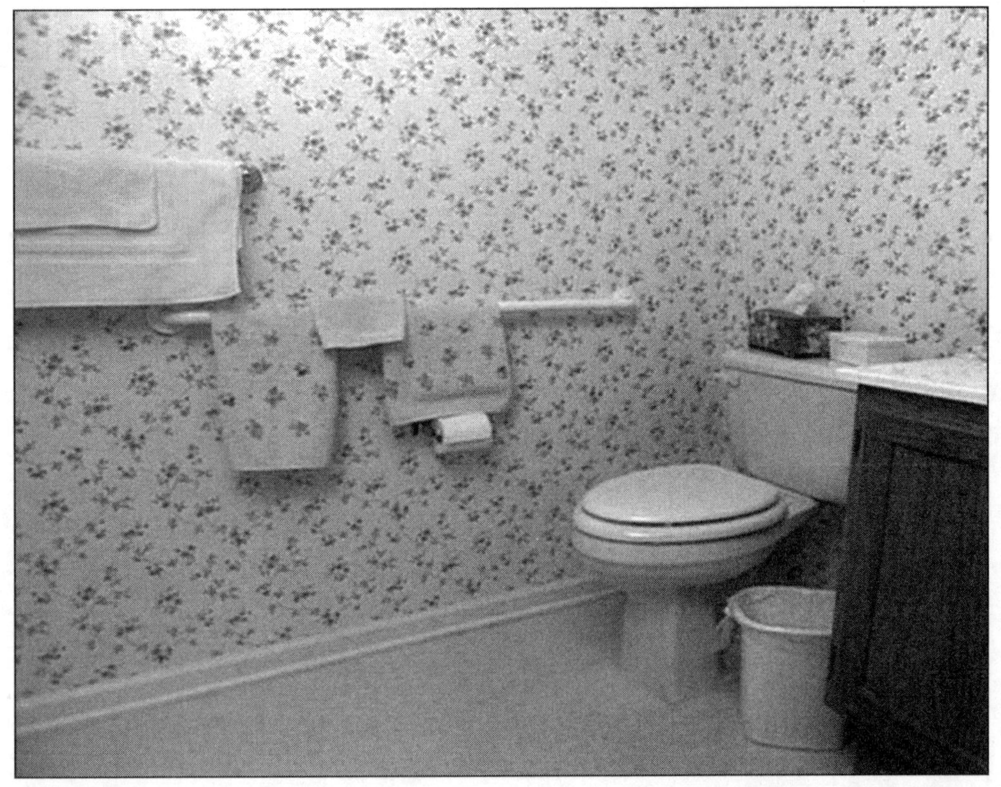

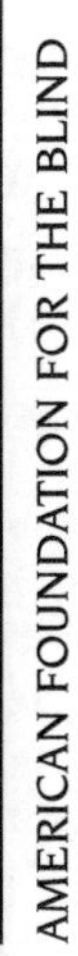

AMERICAN FOUNDATION FOR THE BLIND

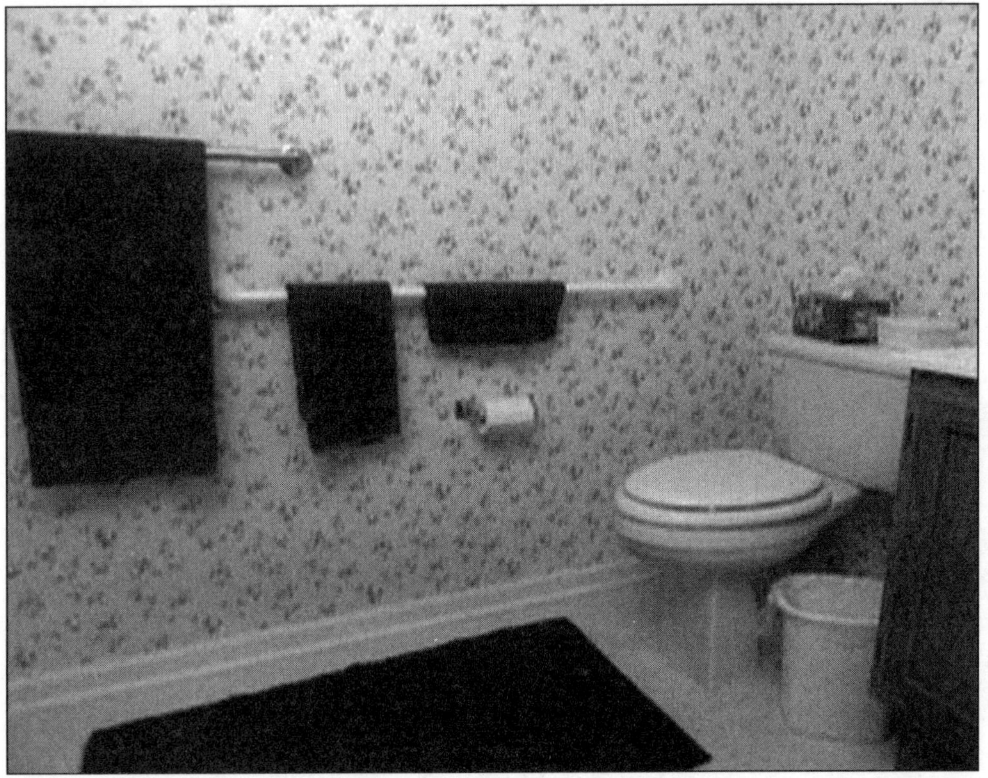

AMERICAN FOUNDATION FOR THE BLIND

Towels with a pattern similar to that of the wallpaper (top) blend in and are difficult to see. Replacing them with dark towels in a color that contrasts with the wall greatly increases their visibility.

SOLUTIONS FOR ENHANCING CONTRAST

Enhancing contrast among elements in the environment is one of the simplest and most effective modifications that you can implement. The difference in light and dark makes objects that contrast with their background easier to see.

You can help the resident in the following ways:

1. Use solid colors as backgrounds to make objects "stand out."
2. Avoid using patterns, prints, or stripes in general.
3. Place light-colored objects against darker backgrounds. For example, a white plate is more visible against a dark-green or navy-blue tablecloth than on white linens.
4. Place dark objects against lighter backgrounds.

To enhance contrast when reading, use black print on nonglossy white, beige, or ivory paper. (For more suggestions, see Appendix C, Tips for Print Readability.)

REDUCED ABILITY TO SEE COLORS

The ability to identify color commonly diminishes with age. Certain eye conditions associated with aging also make it difficult to tell the difference between certain colors.

Colors that are close to each other on the color circle, such as blue and green or red and orange, are most difficult to tell apart. Pastels are also hard to differentiate.

Bright colors are the easiest to see because of their ability to reflect more light. Solid, bright colors, such as red, orange, blue, and green are usually more visible than pastels.

SOLUTIONS FOR REDUCED ABILITY TO SEE COLORS

Using contrasting colors in the environment can make objects more visible; this will help residents identify objects and move about more easily.

For example, it may be difficult for residents to make out exactly where the walls are in a long hallway. Placing a dark-colored railing against light-colored walls can be very effective in enhancing vision.

REDUCED ABILITY TO SEE DEPTH

A decrease in the ability to perceive depth makes it difficult for an individual to determine how close or far away an object is or how high or low something is.

Loss of depth perception makes steps, raised doorsills, and street curbs difficult to recognize and manage. It also makes it difficult to judge the height of a step or a threshold. This increases the risk of the resident tripping or falling.

SOLUTIONS FOR REDUCED DEPTH PERCEPTION

Use color contrast to make it easier to see places where there is a change in level and to judge the height of the change. On stairways, use yellow tape to distinguish the edge of the step. On curbs, use a yellow painted edge.

FLOATERS

Floaters are tiny spots or specks that float across the field of vision. Most people notice them in well-lit rooms or outdoors on a bright day.

SOLUTIONS FOR FLOATERS

There is no definite solution for floaters. Floaters are usually normal, but in some cases they warn of eye problems, such as retinal detachment, especially if they occur with light flashes, and should be checked by an eye care specialist.

DRY EYES

Dry eyes occur when tear glands do not make enough tears or make tears of poor quality. Dry eyes can be uncomfortable, causing itching, burning, or even some loss of vision.

SOLUTIONS FOR DRY EYES

An eye doctor may suggest using a humidifier in the residence or special eyedrops (artificial tears) to help residents with dry eyes. Surgery may be needed for more serious cases of dry eyes.

Congratulations! You have reached the end of Lesson 2. Now go on to the Key Points to review what you have learned in this lesson.

KEY POINTS IN LESSON 2

Normal Changes in the Aging Eye

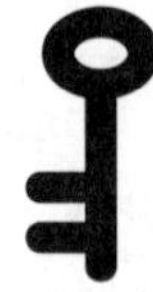

1. Many changes occur in the eye as a result of aging. Although these changes are normal, they affect the overall functioning of individuals as they age.
2. These changes in the eye can result in the following:
   - ➤ inability to focus at close range
   - ➤ inability to see objects clearly
   - ➤ increased need for light
   - ➤ difficulty adapting to dark and light
   - ➤ difficulty with glare
   - ➤ difficulty distinguishing between colors
   - ➤ reduced depth perception

LEARNING ACTIVITIES

Try the following activities to practice what you have learned in this lesson. Some of the activities involve the use of simulators—glasses or similar devices that simulate different types of vision loss. (See Appendix B for sources of vision simulators.) It is important to work in pairs while doing these exercises. One person uses the simulators while the other watches for safety and provides feedback.

Adaptation to dark and light. Put on a pair of simulators that simulate blurred vision. Have someone darken the room. Try to move around. Leave the lights off for a little while and then turn them back on. Try to move around the room.

Write down what you experienced. If you are working with a group, discuss what you experienced.

Reduced depth perception. Wearing the blurred-vision simulators, cover one eye (seeing out of only one eye significantly reduces depth perception). Try to pick up an object. Put the object down on a dark table.

Write down what you experienced. If you are working with a group, discuss what you experienced.

☑ SELF-CHECK

Indicate whether each statement is true (T) or false (F) in the space provided. Check Appendix A for the answers. Then go back and review any statements you may have missed.

______ 1. Glare may make it easier for a person with a visual impairment to distinguish objects.

______ 2. When a person has a problem adapting to dark and light, this is known as reduced depth perception.

______ 3. Contrast is essential for recognizing faces and for reading.

LESSON 3 Eye Conditions Associated with Aging

GOAL

To understand how the major eye conditions or diseases associated with the aging process affect vision and an older person's ability to function independently.

OBJECTIVE

At the end of the lesson, you will be able to describe the types of vision loss experienced by older persons and their functional implications.

Vision Loss in Older People

Although, as explained in Lesson 2, there are various normal changes in vision that occur in the aging eye, there are also a number of eye conditions or diseases that are associated with growing older. For this reason, many older people experience a loss of vision that cannot be corrected with regular eyeglasses.

However, the average older person who is visually impaired is not totally blind. Most people in this category still have some vision but have a *functional vision loss*—that is, their vision loss is severe enough to interfere with their ability to do routine tasks, such as writing a check, reading, cooking, pouring liquids, or using a stove or a microwave. This condition is referred to as *low vision*.

In most cases, older people who have low vision can learn to make the best use of it with specialized instruction and minor adaptations such as the solutions described in Lesson 1.

Types of Vision Loss

THE VISUAL FIELD

The visual field refers to the part of the area around you that you can see when looking straight ahead. This is typically approximately 175 to 180 degrees—nearly a semicircle of the area in front of you. The 180 degrees behind you is never part of the visual field.

Some types of visual impairments involve loss of vision only in certain parts of the visual field, either central vision or side vision. Others cause overall blurring.

LOSS OF CENTRAL VISION

Central vision refers to what you can see right in the middle of your visual field. This is the part of your vision that you use to read and to do other close-up tasks. *Central vision loss* refers to vision loss right in the center of your vision while facing directly ahead of you.

Central vision loss frequently results from one of the leading eye conditions among older people: macular degeneration (which is described in a later section).

Central vision loss makes it difficult to do tasks at a near distance such as

- reading
- doing a handcraft such as sewing
- looking at a photograph

LOSS OF SIDE (PERIPHERAL) VISION

Peripheral vision refers to what you can see from the sides of your eyes while still looking straight ahead. *Peripheral vision loss* refers to vision loss on the side or sides. It creates tunnel vision, similar to what you would see if you looked into a tube or narrow tunnel.

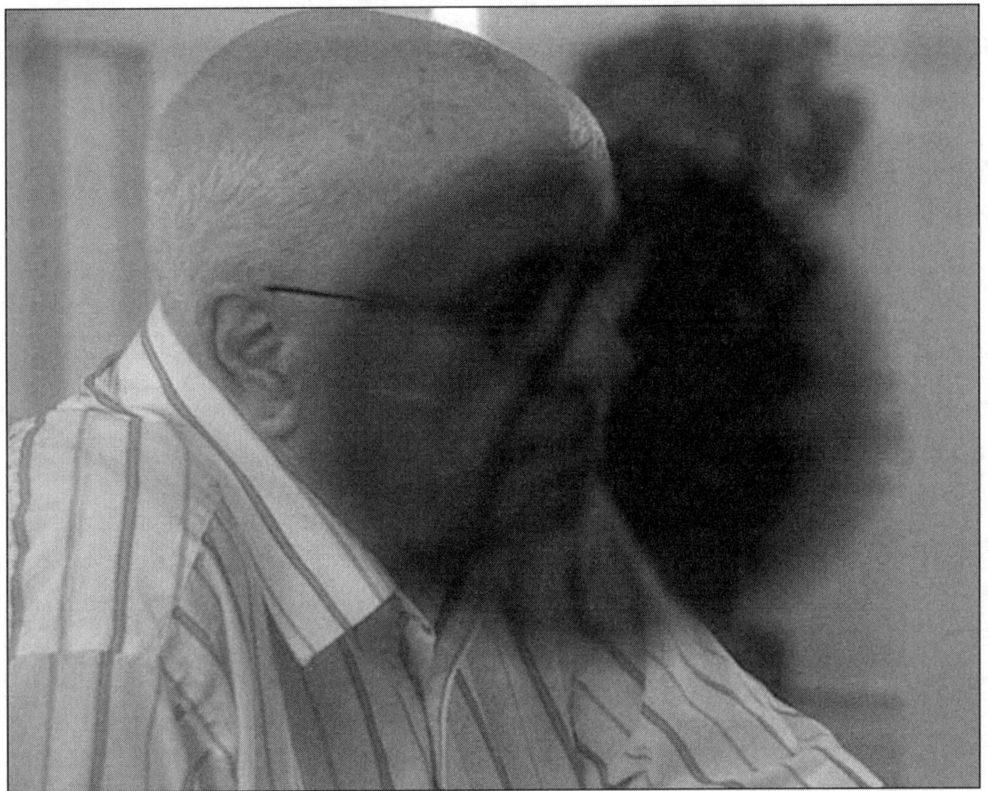

AMERICAN FOUNDATION FOR THE BLIND

Loss of central vision makes it hard to see people's faces and to do things close up, such as reading.

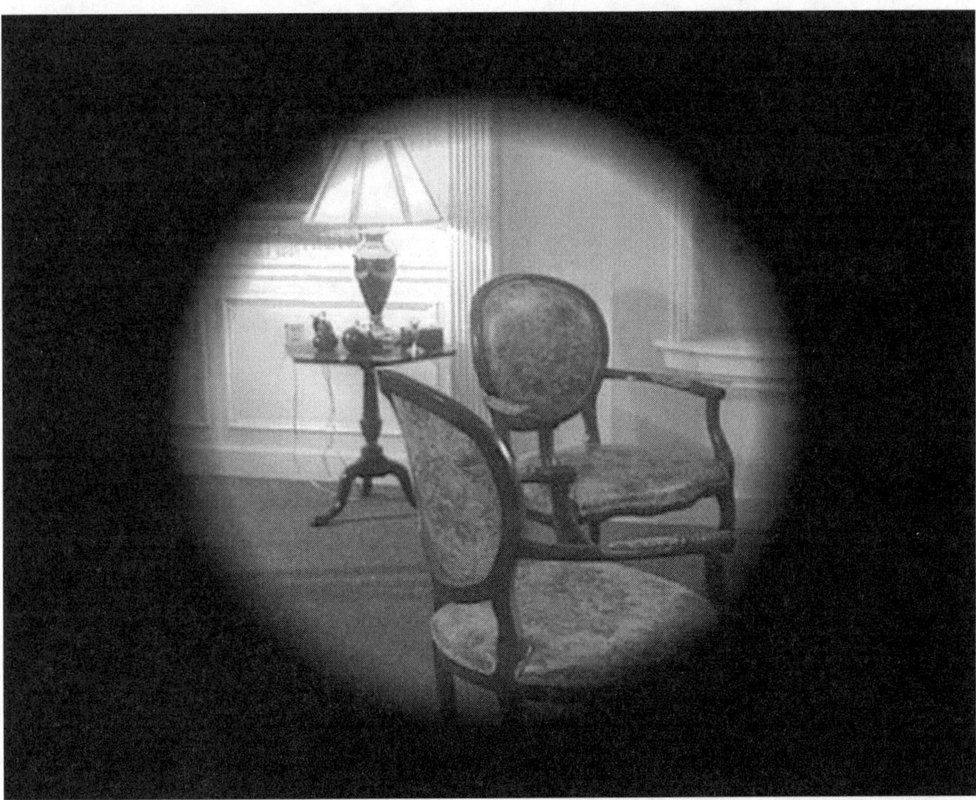

AMERICAN FOUNDATION FOR THE BLIND

Loss of peripheral vision creates tunnel vision, which makes it hard to avoid bumping into objects in the environment.

Peripheral field loss results from eye diseases such as glaucoma (described in later section).

Peripheral vision loss makes moving around more difficult and can result in the following:

- colliding with objects that are off to the side and out of the field of vision
- colliding with objects near the head and out of the field of vision
- colliding with objects by the feet and out of the field of vision

OVERALL BLURRING

Overall blurring refers to seeing everything out of focus. It causes people, objects, and colors to appear hazy and washed out.

Overall blurring can result from diabetic retinopathy, cataracts, or scars on the cornea. (Diabetic retinopathy and cataracts are described in later sections.)

The lack of detail caused by blurred vision makes it difficult to

- read
- tell time
- watch television

Blurred vision also affects depth perception, which may make it difficult to walk safely indoors and outdoors.

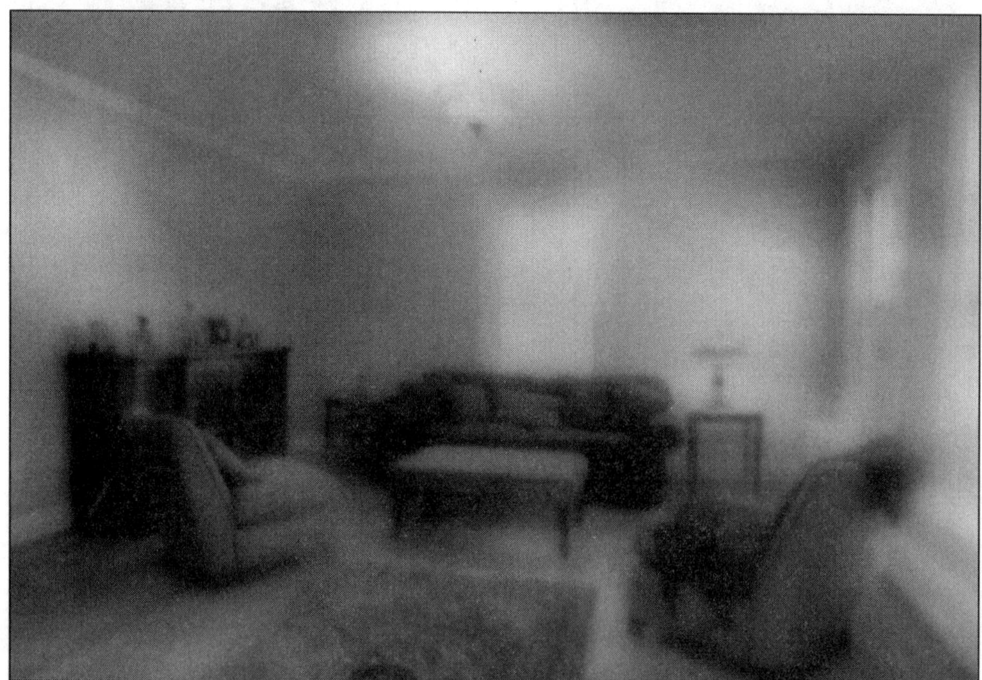

ANDY WARREN

Some forms of vision loss cause overall blurring.

Common Eye Conditions Associated with the Aging Process

Several eye conditions occur more frequently in older people. Although these conditions are associated with aging, they are not part of the normal aging process. The main conditions are covered in the following section. The cross section of the eye (see Figure 3.1) shows the parts of the eye that will be mentioned in the discussions of these eye conditions.

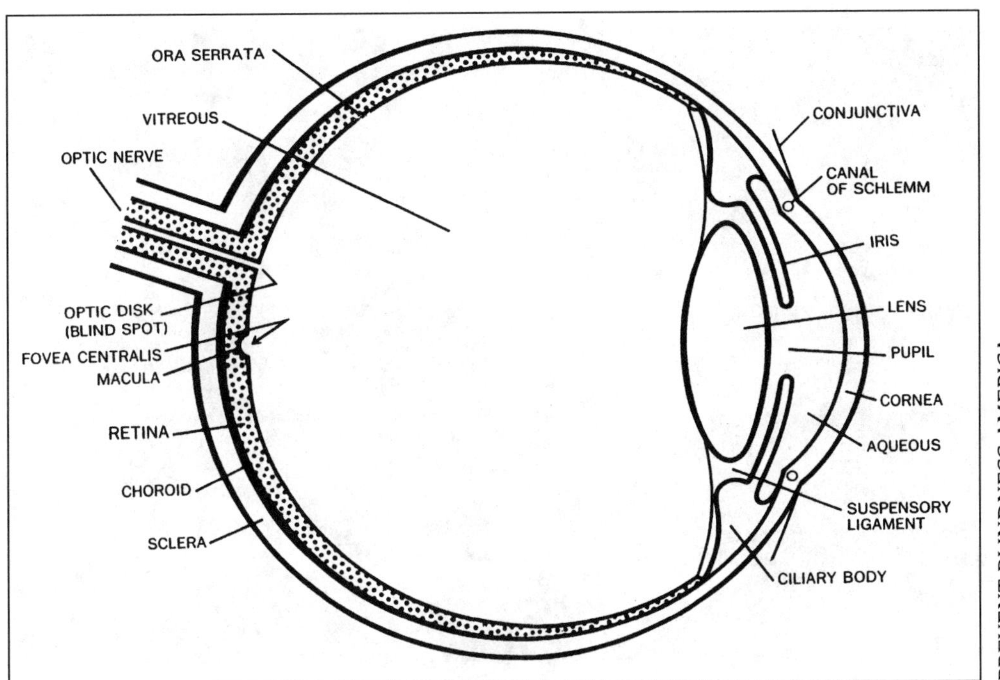

PREVENT BLINDNESS AMERICA

FIGURE 3.1: **CROSS SECTION OF THE EYE.**

MACULAR DEGENERATION

Macular degeneration is the most common eye condition among older people. It weakens the *macula*, which is the central portion of the *retina* (the rear screenlike part of the eye, where the image the eye sees is focused). The macula is the part of the eye responsible for central vision, which is needed to see detail, such as while reading, and for color vision. Macular degeneration results in blurred or distorted central vision and can also result in central blind spots—dark or empty spots or loss of detail vision. Peripheral vision remains intact with macular degeneration.

There are two types of macular degeneration, the "wet" type and the "dry" type. The dry kind most often develops very gradually, but the wet kind can occur quickly. A resident should seek eye medical care right away in the latter case.

What are the symptoms of macular degeneration? Suppose Mrs. O'Brian is a resident with macular degeneration.

- She may see blurry areas on a page.
- She may notice that lines that are straight appear wavy or bent.
- She may mention seeing dark empty spaces in the center of her visual field.

Mrs. O'Brian will still be able to see to the side, or peripherally, unless she has some other eye condition that affects her peripheral vision.

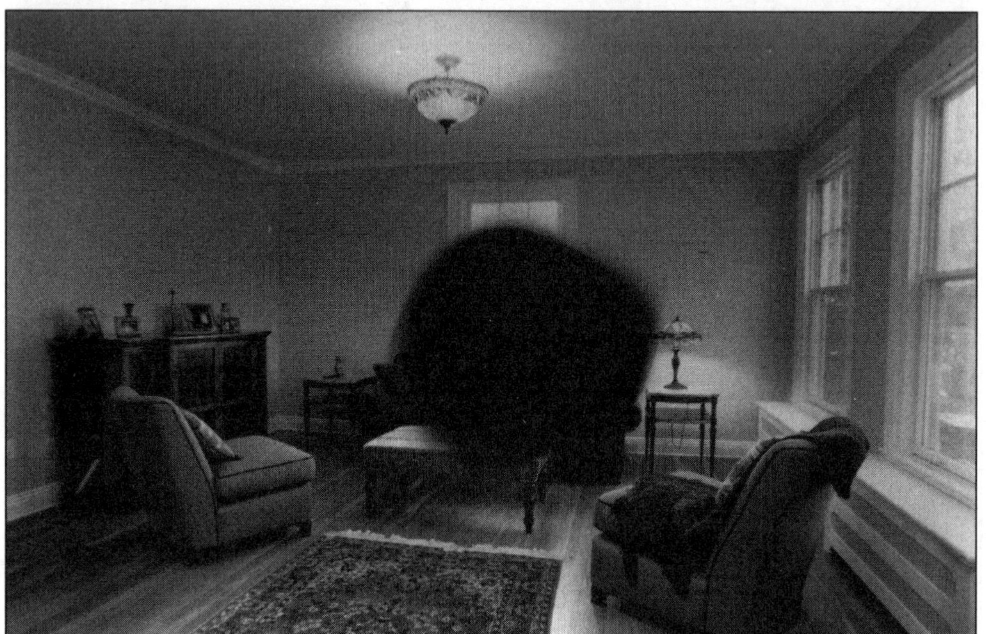

ANDY WARREN

Macular degeneration leaves a blind spot in the middle of the visual field

Mrs. O'Brian may learn *eccentric viewing*, a technique of using peripheral or side vision to see objects. Using side vision moves the blind spot out of the way so that she can see objects that normally would show up in her central field of vision.

Individuals with macular degeneration are often candidates for using special low vision devices to help them see better. (Some of these devices are discussed in Lesson 9.) As her caregiver, you may want to suggest that Mrs. O'Brian have a low vision exam to determine how to make the best use of her remaining vision.

GLAUCOMA

Glaucoma is caused by an increased level of pressure in the eyes (referred to as intraocular pressure) caused by the buildup of excess fluid in the eye. It results in a loss of peripheral or side vision.

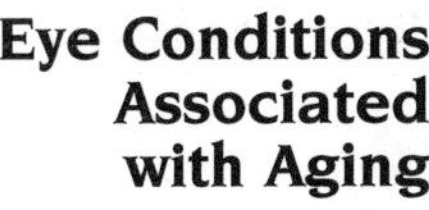

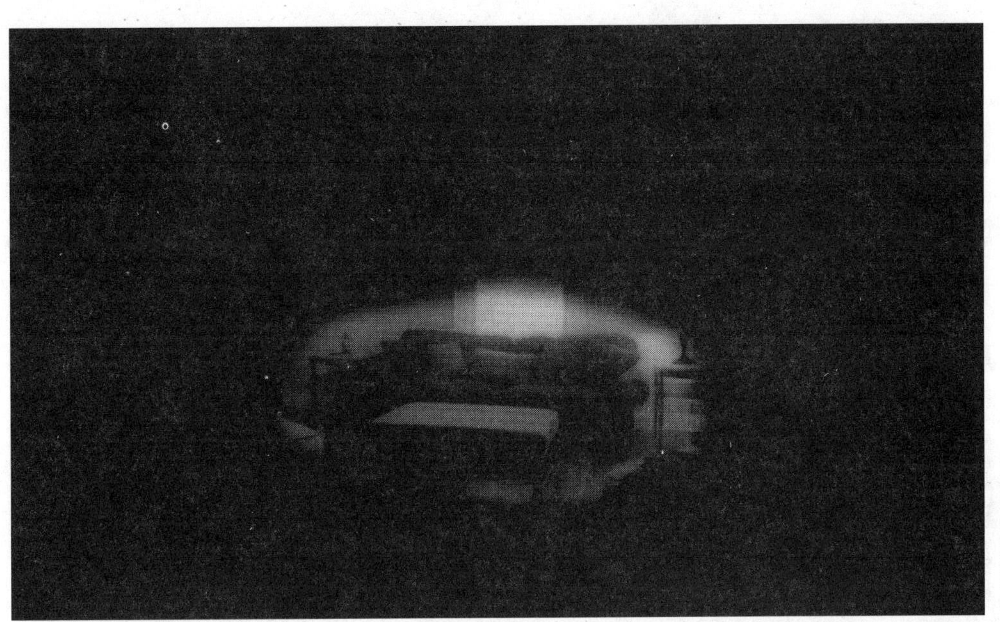

ANDY WARREN

Glaucoma affects side or peripheral vision, causing a tunnel vision effect.

Glaucoma typically affects older people's mobility (ability to move around) because they have trouble detecting objects in the environment.

If it is not diagnosed and treated, chronic elevated eye pressure can cause damage to the *optic nerve* (the nerve that carries the image the eye sees to the brain). Once there is damage to the optic nerve there is nothing that can be done to restore vision. Glaucoma is dangerous because it can occur without symptoms. It is sometimes referred to as the "sneak thief of sight."

Some individuals, such as African-Americans or those with a family history of glaucoma, have a greater risk of developing glaucoma.

How can you tell if a resident may be developing glaucoma? If you notice that Mr. Diaz has started running into objects and doesn't seem to see objects at his side, or if he complains of halos around lights, you need to refer him immediately for medical attention to an eye care specialist. Some forms of glaucoma come on quickly.

There are two types of glaucoma: open-angle and closed-angle glaucoma.

OPEN-ANGLE GLAUCOMA

Open-angle glaucoma occurs when the eye's drainage canals gradually become clogged. This form of glaucoma is slow to affect the vision.

CLOSED-ANGLE GLAUCOMA

Closed-angle glaucoma results from blockage of the angle formed between the iris and the cornea, where fluid normally drains (see

Figure 3.1). This type of glaucoma typically has a sudden, or acute, onset. It is characterized by pain in the eye, blurred vision, nausea, headache, and seeing rainbows around lights at night. A resident with these symptoms needs immediate medical attention from an eye care specialist.

DIABETIC RETINOPATHY

Diabetic retinopathy occurs when small blood vessels in the eye stop feeding the retina. In the early stages of the disease, the blood vessels may leak fluid in the retina, which can affect the macula, the entire retina, or the *vitreous* (the clear, gellike substance that fills the interior of the eye). This leaking fluid distorts vision. It can cause overall blurring or scattered blind spots and can also affect peripheral vision.

Diabetic retinopathy is associated with diabetes, both type I and type II. Diabetes can cause cataracts and glaucoma. Older people with high blood pressure and poor control of blood sugar levels are more likely to lose vision from retinopathy. Controlling a resident's blood sugar levels and high blood pressure may slow the progression of diabetic eye disease, but it will not necessarily prevent it.

Individuals who are Hispanic, African-American, or Native American have a higher risk of developing diabetes. You should be

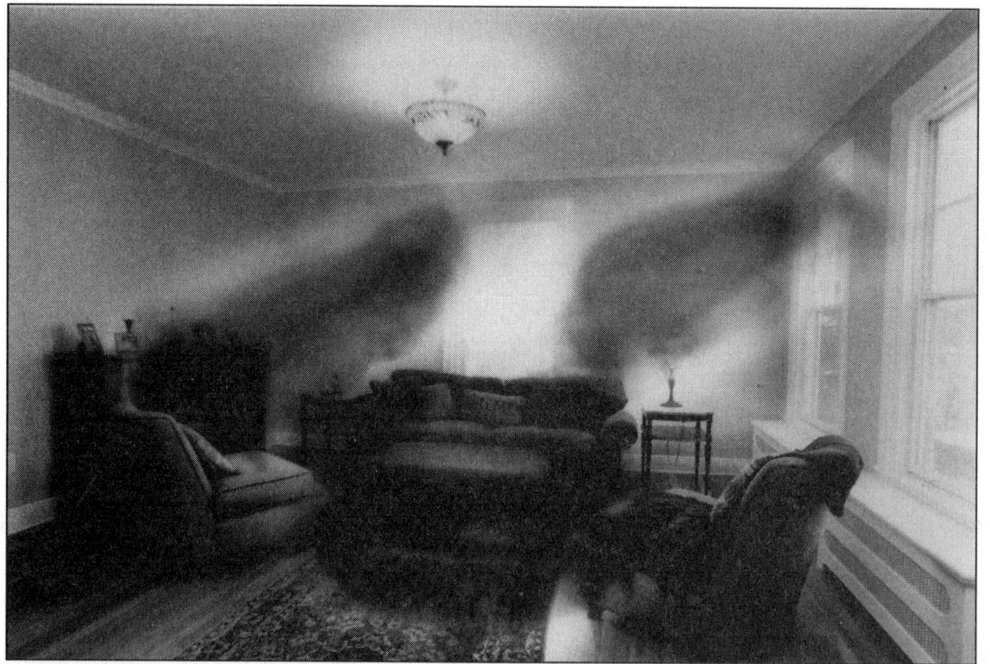

ANDY WARREN

Diabetic retinopathy can cause scattered blind spots or overall blurring (as shown on the next page).

aware that residents in these ethnic groups, or any residents with diabetes, should have routine medical and eye care at regular intervals, at least annually or more often as prescribed by a doctor. If, for example, Mrs. Garcia, a resident who has not been tested for diabetes, experiences a sudden loss of vision, she should see her eye care specialist immediately.

CATARACTS

Cataracts are cloudy areas in the lens of the eye. Whereas a healthy lens is clear and lets light through it, cataracts prevent light from passing easily through the lens. This results in loss of vision and overall blurriness in vision.

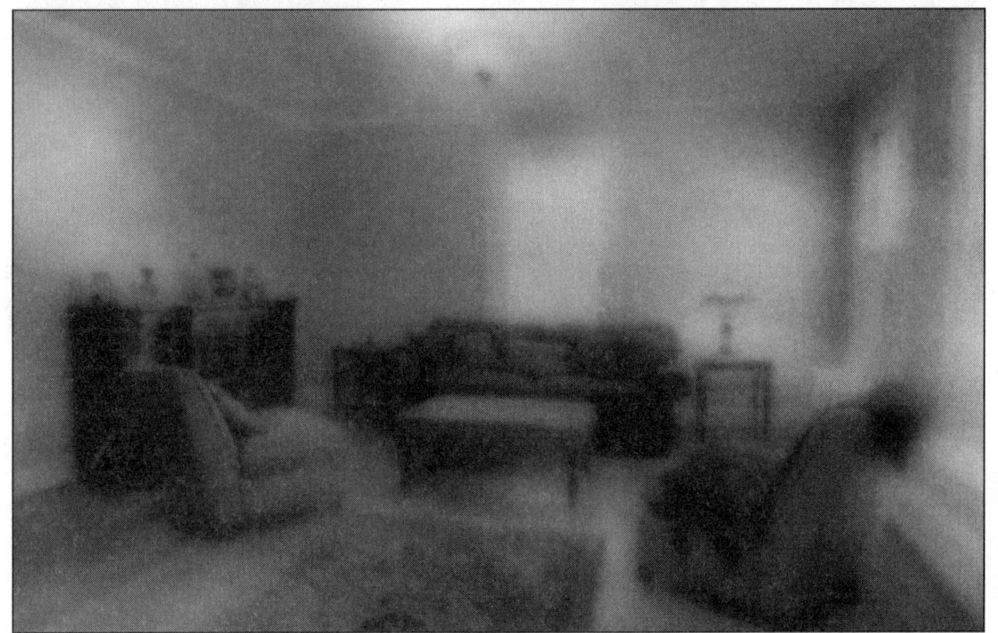

ANDY WARREN

Cataracts cause overall blurring and haziness of vision.

As the lens of the eye ages in most people, the center of the lens turns yellow and loses its ability to focus on close tasks. It eventually turns amber and then brown, letting in less and less light.

Most cataracts form slowly and cause no pain, redness, or tearing in the eye. Cataracts can be treated successfully by surgery 95 percent of the time, usually in an outpatient facility.

How can you tell if a resident may be developing cataracts? If you notice that Mrs. DeCarlo is beginning to shield her eyes more and more from glare and complains about her vision getting hazier, you may want to suggest that she have an eye exam. She may have cataracts or some other eye disease with similar symptoms.

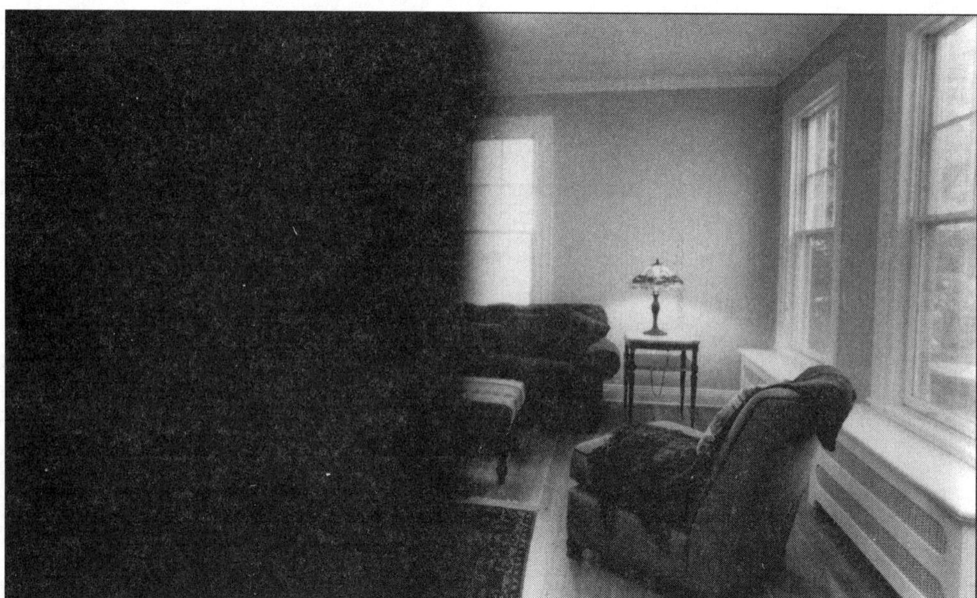

ANDY WARREN

Hemianopia, or loss of vision in half the visual field, can result from a cerebral stroke.

HEMIANOPIA

Hemianopia is vision loss in half of the visual field as a result of a cerebral stroke. The type of vision loss depends on the area of the brain involved in the stroke.

In working with Mr. Thomas, a resident who has had a stroke, you need to be aware that hemianopia in either brain hemisphere can affect reading. Mr. Thomas, a resident with hemianopia, will have difficulty finding the beginning of lines of text if vision loss is on the left side; it may be difficult to see the ends of words if vision loss is on the right side.

He may consistently bump into objects on the affected side. He may also have problems putting on his clothes and many other activities. He must learn to make good use of remaining vision associated with the unaffected hemisphere of his brain.

Mr. Thomas may also benefit from a low vision exam and may be helped by the prescription of a special prism lens which can help him use his vision in the unaffected side of his brain.

COMBINED EYE DISORDERS

It is also possible to experience several of these eye disorders at the same time, such as glaucoma and cataracts, macular degeneration and diabetic retinopathy, or cataracts, glaucoma, and diabetic retinopathy. In most cases, medical and surgical interventions are only effective in stopping or slowing the progression of the disorder. They usually cannot restore vision that has already been lost or damaged, although surgery is usually effective in removing cataracts.

Assessing Residents for Vision Loss

Because you work with residents every day, you are in a good position to notice any signs of change in their vision and to take note of any symptoms that they report.

SIGNS AND SYMPTOMS OF VISION LOSS

It is important for professionals, paraprofessionals (such as personal care aides), volunteers, and family members of residents to be able to recognize signs of vision loss. It is particularly important to notice early warnings of a sudden loss of vision so that the older person can be referred to an eye care professional for immediate eye medical care. The resident might also benefit from vision rehabilitation services that can help him or her learn new, adaptive ways of doing routine tasks.

Some of the symptoms of vision loss that the resident may report are listed below.

SYMPTOMS OF VISION LOSS

- sudden hazy or blurred vision
- recurrent pain in or around the eyes
- double vision
- seeing flashes of light
- seeing halos around lights
- unusual sensitivity to light or glare
- changes in the color of the iris
- sudden development of persisting floaters (particles in the vitreous fluid in the back portion of the eye)

When working with the residents in your care, you will often be in a position to notice other signs that a resident may be gradually losing some vision, such as problems carrying out daily living tasks that the resident has normally done independently. You can assess the resident informally in two ways: by asking a few simple nonthreatening questions and by observing the resident.

INQUIRE

If you suspect that Mr. Casey has lost some of his vision, you can ask him a few questions, without frightening him, that can reveal whether he may be having trouble with his eyesight, such as

- Are you having any difficulty reading that book?
- Are you having any trouble recognizing faces?

OBSERVE

Signs that Mr. Casey may be losing his vision can be observed while he is doing routine tasks such as reading and writing, moving about in the environment, or eating and drinking.

SIGNS OF VISION LOSS

- stopping uncertainly
- hesitant steps
- shuffling feet
- underreaching (not reaching far enough) when picking up objects
- overreaching (reaching too far) when picking up objects

For more information on signs of vision loss and what to do if you notice them, see Appendix D, How to Recognize Vision Loss in Older People.

It is important to report the situation to your supervisor or the proper person on staff if Mr. Casey shows any signs of difficulty with his everyday activities, such as reading, writing, eating, pursuing normal recreational activities, or personal hygiene.

Eye Care and Vision-Related Services

If Mr. Casey may have an eye problem or vision loss, it is important to get help for him from the appropriate eye care professional. There are different kinds of services for people who have visual impairments, which are offered by several different professionals.

MEDICAL EYE CARE

There are two types of medical eye care professionals: *optometrists* and *ophthalmologists*. Both can conduct a thorough eye examination, perform examinations on dilated eyes, and prescribe eyeglasses and needed medications. Ophthalmologists can also perform surgery on the eye.

LOW VISION ASSESSMENT

A *low vision assessment* is different from an eye medical examination. A low vision assessment is a complete evaluation of how the person uses his or her vision. It covers the person's visual impairment and visual ability and the possibilities for making use of his or her remaining sight. The examination finds out whether special low vision devices can help the person make better use of his or her vision. (See Lessons 9 and 10 for more information on low vision devices.) Both optometrists and ophthalmologists who have special training in low vision can provide this service.

VISION REHABILITATION SERVICES

Another professional, known as a *rehabilitation teacher,* teaches people with visual impairments adapted ways of performing their everyday activities (as described in the lessons throughout this manual). If a resident needs or expresses an interest in more instruction than a staff member can provide using this manual, a staff member should make a referral to a local agency or state agency that serves individuals who are blind or visually impaired. (For a listing of such services, see Appendix G, Independent Living Services for Older Individuals Who Are Blind.)

Limited funds are available from the federal Independent Living Services for Older Individuals Who Are Blind program to help qualified older people pay for training in independent living skills and for adaptive equipment. Some states use these funds to provide a low vision assessment, and most provide training by an orientation and mobility specialist on how to move about safely outdoors using a white cane.

Congratulations! You have reached the end of Lesson 3. Now go on to the Key Points to review what you have learned in this lesson.

KEY POINTS IN LESSON 3

Overview of Vision Loss

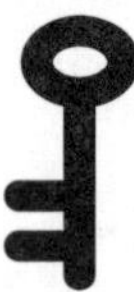

1. Age-related eye conditions can result in three types of vision loss:
   - loss of central vision
   - loss of side (peripheral) vision
   - overall blurring
2. The major eye conditions associated with aging are
   - macular degeneration
   - glaucoma
   - diabetic retinopathy
   - cataracts
   - hemianopia resulting from a stroke
3. There are several signs of vision loss that you should be aware of, including sudden hazy or blurred vision and pain around the eyes.
4. It may be necessary to refer the resident to an eye care specialist, a low vision specialist, and a vision rehabilitation agency for further evaluation and assistance.

LEARNING ACTIVITIES

Try the following activities to practice what you have learned in this lesson. Some of the activities involve the use of simulators—glasses that simulate different types of vision loss. (See Appendix B for sources of vision simulators.) It is important to work in pairs while doing these exercises. One person uses the simulators while the other watches for safety and provides feedback.

Using the simulators for each of the different types of vision loss, try

- eating a meal
- walking around (particularly in an area with glare)
- pouring water into a glass
- identifying money

- ➤ dialing a phone
- ➤ another activity that you and your partner decide on

O-π Discuss the results of this activity with other staff. How can you use your experiences to help residents with visual impairments?

O-π Identify residents with as many of the major eye conditions as possible and describe the signs or behaviors observed that indicate the presence of an eye condition.

☑ SELF-CHECK

Indicate whether each statement is true (T) or false (F) in the space provided. Check Appendix A for the answers. Then go back and review any statements you may have missed.

______ 1. Loss of central vision means a person may have a hard time seeing my face or reading regular print.

______ 2. Loss of side vision means a person may have a hard time seeing things in the center of vision.

______ 3. A resident who begins to have trouble getting around his or her room or begins to have trouble recognizing people is probably just depressed and should be left alone.

______ 4. Different types of visual impairments affect people in different ways.

LESSON 4 Assessing the Environment

GOALS

- To evaluate a resident's room as well as common areas to identify any possible obstacles or hazards for a person who is visually impaired.
- To find ways to modify the environment to help a visually impaired resident get around more safely and independently.

OBJECTIVES

At the end of the lesson you will be able to

- evaluate a resident's room and common areas
- identify needed changes in the environment
- maximize the safety and independence of a resident who is visually impaired

Assessing the Environment for Safety

It is extremely important to ensure the safety of all residents. This is even more important for residents who are visually impaired. A person who is visually impaired may have a slower reaction time and may be more prone to encountering hazards than others.

You can help make the facility, program, and activities safer and more accessible for residents by making a few simple changes to the environment. It is not necessarily expensive or complicated. Before making any changes, though, you need to know about the common hazards and the possible solutions. These involve lighting, color contrast, and glare reduction.

Remember that the changes you suggest will help all residents, not just those with age-related eye conditions. As explained in Lesson 2, because of normal changes in the eye, almost all older people need more light to see well and have reduced visual acuity and less sensitivity to contrast. Keep this in mind as you conduct the assessment.

The first step to determining what changes may be needed in the environment is conducting an *environmental assessment* using the environmental checklist in Appendix F. You will need to walk through the resident's room and all the common areas of the facility to see where there may be problems and what the solutions to them may be. This assessment should be conducted using simulators so that you can "see" the environment from the perspective of the resident with a visual impairment. Try out all the simulators so that you can understand how residents with a variety of eye conditions have to function in the facility. The results of the assessment should be shared with your supervisor.

The important things to look for in your environmental assessment are hazards, lighting, glare, color, and contrast.

QUESTIONS TO ASK IN AN ENVIRONMENTAL ASSESSMENT

- Are there **obstacles** or **hazards** that the resident might encounter?
- Is the **lighting** good enough?
- Is there **glare** that can make it harder for the resident to see?
- Are bright **colors** and **contrast** used to make the environment and the objects in it more visible?

These questions are discussed in the following sections.

Safety First

The first thing to check for when examining the resident's environment are obstacles or hazards that are often found in facilities where older persons with visual impairments live, such as the ones listed here.

HAZARDS

- **Doors** or **cabinet doors** left ajar rather than completely closed or completely open are a potential hazard. It is easy for a resident with a visual impairment to run into them.
- **Furniture** moved from its regular location can create an unsafe situation.
- **Floor coverings** that are slick and have a great deal of glare are potentially dangerous, as are area rugs that do not have a nonstick surface.
- **Doorsills** are a major cause of falls because it is very easy for an older person to trip over them.
- **Glare** on highly polished floors or on tabletops makes it very difficult for visually impaired residents to see.

SOLUTIONS

- Doors should be kept completely open or completely closed. Closet and cabinet doors should be kept closed.
- The edges of rugs and corners should be tacked and/or taped down. Small area rugs may be removed or tacked down. Worn and torn carpeting and linoleum should be removed.
- Potentially slippery floors can be covered with a textured runner or carpeting that is secured. Likewise, a floor runner that is secured can provide needed contrast against a textured floor covering. A solid-color floor covering is less confusing for older residents with vision loss than one with a pattern.
- Doorsills should be reduced to no more than one quarter inch for safety. Using a contrasting color for the doorsill is also useful.

Solutions to glare are covered in a later section of this lesson.

Lighting

Good and appropriate lighting is one of the most important factors in making the resident's environment safer and easier to get around. You need to understand the full impact lighting can have on the resident who is experiencing age-related vision loss. For example, limited lighting would make it difficult to nearly impossible to read or move around safely in the environment.

There are six types of light. The following is a summary of the characteristics of each type.

TYPES OF LIGHT

TYPE OF LIGHT	CHARACTERISTICS	USE
sunlight	full-spectrum natural light	best overall, can create glare
incandescent lighting	standard lightbulbs	best for close tasks
full-spectrum lightbulbs	lightbulbs such as Chromalux, close to natural sunlight	brighter and cleaner than incandescent
fluorescent lighting	less bright, less focused light, flickers	good for general room lighting
combination incandescent and fluorescent lighting	multiple light sources or combined in one fixture	combination is best for most everyday activities
halogen light	bright, focused, very hot	requires special precautions

SUNLIGHT

Sunlight is the best, most natural type of light. It is good for both indoor and outdoor activities. Sunlight is a full-spectrum light; that is, it contains all the colors of light (red, orange, yellow, green, blue, indigo, and violet) in equal amounts, which makes it easier for individuals with visual impairment to see.

However, sunlight can create outdoor and indoor glare. Sunlight can produce glare on shiny surfaces such as polished floors or tabletops, which can then interfere with functioning.

INCANDESCENT LIGHTING

Incandescent lighting, found in standard lightbulbs, is very concentrated and very stable. It does not flicker. It is best for concentrated lighting on close work, such as reading, sewing, and other close-up tasks.

Incandescent lighting is best when used in table lamps and swing-arm or gooseneck fixtures. It is not appropriate for general room lighting because it can cause shadowy spots and glare.

Higher wattages (such as 100-watt bulbs) can be helpful in producing brighter light, but they also produce more heat, making them inappropriate for prolonged close work.

FULL-SPECTRUM LIGHTBULBS

Full-spectrum lightbulbs, such as Chromalux, produce light that is closer to natural sunlight than are regular incandescent bulbs, and the light is brighter and cleaner. These bulbs can be used in any fixture in which a regular incandescent bulb is used.

FLUORESCENT LIGHTING

Fluorescent lighting is not bright enough for close work like reading, needlework, or crafts. It is not stable and can flicker, producing a "strobe" effect. However, fluorescent bulbs light a wider area than incandescents and do not create shadowy spots or glare.

There are now compact fluorescent lamps (CFLs) that fit into regular lamp sockets and provide illumination that is comparable to incandescent light. These produce less heat and use less energy.

COMBINATION INCANDESCENT AND FLUORESCENT LIGHTING

Combination incandescent and fluorescent lighting is usually the most useful and comfortable light for most everyday activities. The combination of incandescent and fluorescent light creates a full-spectrum light, the closest to natural sunlight. Incandescent light fills in the gaps in the fluorescent spectrum.

Throughout the facility, try to combine fluorescent and incandescent lighting whenever possible. Use fluorescents or CFLs for general room lighting. Supplement them with incandescent bulbs in adjustable swing-arm desk and floor lamps for task lighting.

It is possible to combine fluorescent and incandescent lighting in the same fixture. Some adjustable swing-arm lamps contain a fluorescent "ring" that surrounds an incandescent lightbulb.

HALOGEN LAMPS

Some individuals prefer halogen light because it is brighter, "whiter," more concentrated, and more energy-efficient than incandescent light. It is used in lamps, track lighting, and recessed ceiling fixtures, and is also available in adjustable swing-arm lamps.

Be aware that halogen light is hotter and more focused and requires a shield to use. It produces intense heat and can cause fire, severe burns, or other personal injury if used incorrectly. It is not recommended, therefore, for prolonged close work, such as reading, knitting, sewing, or crafts.

Always follow the manufacturer's safety precautions when using halogen light. Halogen lighting is not allowed in facilities in some states due to the potential hazard it poses.

Glare

Glare is reflected or uncontrolled light in the environment that shines directly into the eyes and causes physical discomfort and/or reduces visual clarity. Glare can interfere with a resident's visual comfort, physical safety, or ability to peform many activities independently.

Sensitivity to glare often results from the combination of age-related vision changes and eye conditions such as cataracts and diabetic retinopathy, as discussed in Lessons 2 and 3. Glare can be caused by

- uncontrolled sunlight on highly polished tile or wood floors
- shiny tabletops and wall coverings
- chrome fixtures and mirrors in the bathroom
- uncovered lightbulbs
- windows without curtains or shades in hallways, dining rooms, and reception areas

Glare can be reduced by controlling the source of light or covering the reflective surface.

- Use miniblinds to control the amount of direct sunlight in a room.

- Use a nonskid area rug to alleviate glare on a highly polished floor.
- Use a tablecloth to reduce glare on a shining tabletop.
- Cover lightbulbs with a shade to reduce glare.
- Use dark towels and washcloths to reduce the reflection from a mirror and stainless steel or porcelain fixtures to reduce glare in the bathroom.

Color and Contrast

Color and contrast are key elements in the environment. Use of bright and contrasting colors makes surroundings and objects easier to see. For example, it can make a program activity accessible to residents who are visually impaired and allow them to participate independently in recreational and leisure activities.

COLOR

Brightness is an important characteristic of color. Bright colors are easiest to see because they reflect the most light. Solid bright colors such as red and orange are more visible than pastel colors.

Color can be used to help provide a resident with important safety information such as

- warning of a change in the surface in the floor
- warning of steps, construction, or other hazards
- identification of different areas through color coding (for example, yellow for the dining room, blue for rest rooms, and red for activity areas)

COLOR CONTRAST

Increasing contrast between an object and its background makes the object easier to see. The following tips will help you use contrast to make objects more visible in the environment:

- Solid colors as background make objects stand out.
- When choosing backgrounds, such as the walls and floors, avoid prints, patterns, and stripes. Solid bright colors are the easiest to see.
- Place light-colored objects against darker backgrounds to make them stand out; place dark objects against lighter backgrounds.

To promote safety and independence for residents, ask yourself, "Is contrast being used effectively in this room?" as you assess your facility's environment. Share your findings with your supervisor or other appropriate staff person.

For additional information about improving the environment for older persons with visual impairments, see Appendix E, Creating a Functional Environment for Older People Who Are Visually Impaired.

Congratulations! You have reached the end of Lesson 4. Now go on to the Key Points to review what you have learned in this lesson.

KEY POINTS IN LESSON 4

Assessing the Resident's Environment

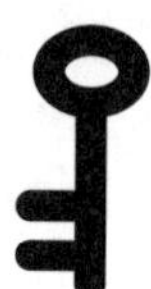

1. To ensure the safety of residents, it is important to assess the facility and remove hazards.
   - Remove hazards such as throw rugs.
   - Make sure doors are kept completely closed or completely open.
   - Make sure floors are not slippery.
   - Reduce glare in the resident's room and in hallways and public areas.
   - Use appropriate lighting.
   - Return furniture to its usual place.
2. Assess the facility for best use of contrast, lighting, and glare reduction to enhance the resident's ability to move around in the facility.
3. Most older people experience some degree of vision changes and can benefit from environmental modifications.

LEARNING ACTIVITIES

Try the following activities to practice what you have learned in this lesson. Some of the activities involve the use of simulators—glasses that simulate different types of vision loss. (See Appendix B for sources of vision simulators.) It is important to work in pairs while doing these exercises. One person uses the simulators while the other watches for safety and provides feedback.

- Ask someone to move the furniture around in the training room or dining area. If possible, open the curtains to allow maximum sunlight. Put on a set of the simulators and try to move around in the room.
- Place a table next to a window with a great deal of glare. Put on a set of the simulators. Try eating from a white plate on a white tablecloth. Then reduce the glare by closing the curtains or blinds. Substitute a dark plate and napkin for the white plate. Try eating.
- Using a set of simulators, try walking down a hallway that faces a window with glare created by sunlight.
- Using a set of the simulators, go into a bathroom with all white fixtures and white towels. Try washing your hands and locating a towel.

SELF-CHECK

Indicate whether each statement is true (T) or false (F) in the space provided. Check Appendix A for the answers. Then go back and review any statements you may have missed.

_______ 1. A resident who has a visual impairment should be seated at a dining room table that faces the sun.

_______ 2. Lighting and color contrast are two important factors to check when assessing the resident's environment.

_______ 3. It is recommended that area rugs be used throughout the facility.

LESSON 5

Getting Around the Environment

GOAL

To enable you to help the older resident move around safely and confidently in the environment.

OBJECTIVE

At the end of this lesson, you will be able to teach the resident the skills necessary to get around her environment safely, efficiently, and confidently.

TEACH Principles

When working with a resident to help him or her get around in her environment, use the five TEACH principles for working successfully with a resident who is visually impaired:

T—Talk to the resident about what you are teaching him or her to do.

E—Encourage the resident to try the techniques in this lesson.

A—Assess the resident's ability to move around independently in the environment.

C—"Can do" is the motto for each resident.

H—Help the resident to learn the techniques he or she wishes to use to get around the environment.

Helping a Resident Get Around the Facility

You may be asked to help a resident with a visual impairment get around the facility; for example, from the resident's room to the dining hall or activity room. This lesson will teach you certain techniques that will help you with this task.

> **CAUTION:** Mobility instructors are specially trained to teach persons who are blind or visually impaired to get around safely and efficiently in their environment. Residents who need more than a simple orientation to their environment or who are interested in using a white cane to move about should be referred to a local vision rehabilitation agency for more training by an orientation and mobility specialist.

Sighted Guide Technique

Sighted guide is a method of walking with and guiding a person who is blind or visually impaired safely and efficiently. In this technique, you act as the guide and ask the resident to take your arm and let you guide him or her. The visually impaired person will follow the movements of your body as you walk. This is safer than taking hold of the resident and attempting to pull or push him or her in front of you.

There are several different aspects to the sighted guide technique in addition to the basic technique for walking. These include moving through a narrow space, going through a doorway, going up and down stairs, sitting down, and getting into a car. Use the photographs to follow along with the descriptions of the techniques. When you guide a resident you also need to be aware of the environment.

The following are the steps for walking with a resident using the basic sighted guide technique.

WALKING WITH A RESIDENT

STEP 1 When preparing to walk with a resident who is visually impaired, always ask if he or she wants assistance.

STEP 2 Touch the resident's hand with the back of your hand to communicate that you are there. Advise the resident to take your arm just above your elbow. For more support, she may need to grasp your forearm as well.

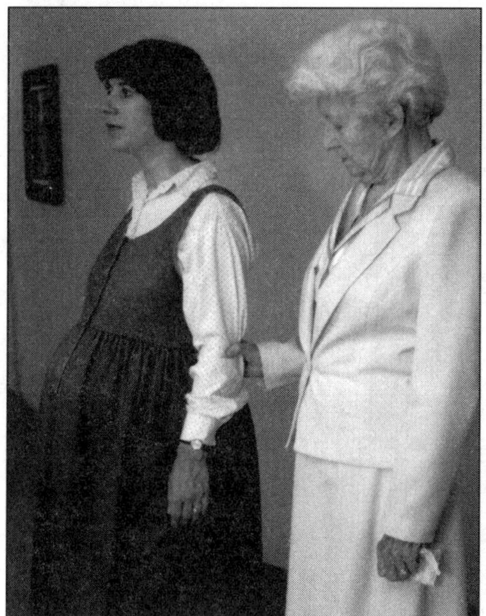

In the basic sighted guide technique, the resident grasps the sighted guide's arm just above the elbow. She walks one-half step behind and slightly to the side.

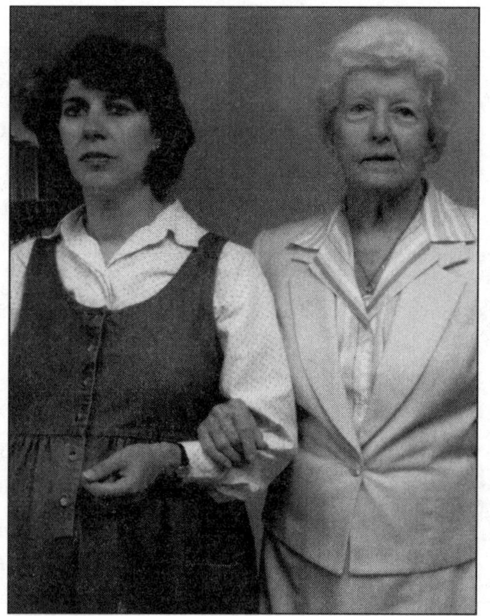

An older resident may need to use an alternate technique for extra support, such as grasping the forearm of the sighted guide. In that case, she will have to walk alongside the guide.

ANN G. HUBBARD

STEP 3 Ask the resident to walk about one-half step behind you and a little to the side. In that way, the resident can follow the motion of your body as you walk. If you are using the more supportive method, in which the resident takes hold of your forearm, he or she should be at your side.

STEP 4 Walk at a comfortable pace, adjusting your pace to the resident's comfort level.

STEP 5 As you walk, talk to the resident and explain where you are going. Tell the resident if you are coming to the end of a hallway or if you have to veer to avoid an object in the path, such as a medication cart. The more descriptive you can be, the more confident the resident will feel.

When you have to walk through a space that is too narrow for you and the resident to pass through in the basic sighted guide position, you need to adjust the technique.

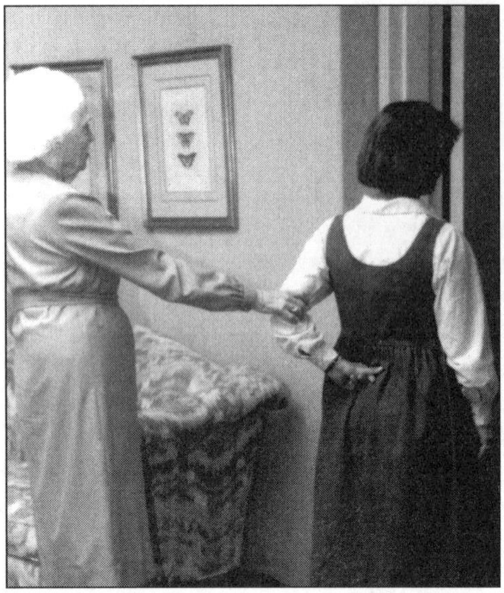

ANN G. HUBBARD

When guiding a resident through a narrow space, place your arm behind your back and have the resident walk directly behind you.

GOING THROUGH A NARROW SPACE

STEP 1 When guiding a resident through a narrow space, be sure to talk to the resident. Explain that you have to go through a narrow space and that the resident must walk behind you.

STEP 2 Move the arm that the resident is holding so that your hand is behind your back and you are guiding the resident to walk directly behind you. At the same time tell the resident to move behind you. In this way, both of you can go through the narrow space one after the other.

STEP 3 After you have passed through the narrow space, return your arm to the basic sighted guide position. This will bring the resident back to his or her position walking one-half step behind you.

If the resident is unable to carry out this technique, have the resident stand behind you and put his or her arm around your waist for more support. You may need to turn to one side and face the resident. This way you can sidestep through the space together.

Going through a doorway while guiding a resident requires another modification of the basic technique.

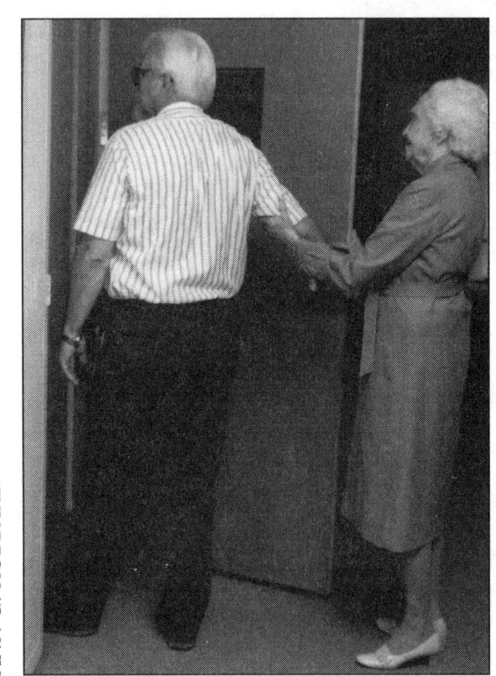

ANN G. HUBBARD

When walking though a doorway, have the resident hold the door open with her free hand while you both walk through.

GOING THROUGH A DOORWAY

STEP 1 When guiding a resident to go through a doorway, talk to the resident. Explain that you are approaching a door and tell whether the door is opening toward you or away from you.

STEP 2 It may be necessary for the resident to change sides with you to go through the door safely and efficiently. The resident should be on the side closest to the door hinges. Ask the resident to move behind you as if going through a narrow passage way. Ask the resident to continue grasping your arm while reaching for your other arm. The resident should grip the other arm in a sighted guide position. (Continuing to maintain contact is safer and less disorienting for the resident.) The resident can then release the hold on the initial arm and maintain the sighted guide position with the other arm.

STEP 3 Ask the resident to walk behind you as you do when going through a narrow space.

STEP 4 Open the door and ask the resident to hold the door with the other hand while both of you go through.

If the resident is unable to hold the door, you may have to open the door, hold it and gently guide the resident through while supporting him or her.

It is always important to alert the resident you are guiding to any changes in the level or surface of the floor. If it is necessary to guide a resident on a stairway, use the following technique.

WALKING UP OR DOWN STAIRS

STEP 1 When guiding a resident on a stairway, talk to the resident. Explain which way the steps are going—up or down—and how many steps there are.

STEP 2 Position the resident so that he or she can grab the handrail. Make sure the resident is approaching the stairway straight on, not at an angle.

STEP 3 Walk up or down the steps in front of the resident. Pause to tell the resident when you come to a landing and to the last step.

When you are guiding a resident who is ready to sit down, it is important to make sure the resident knows where he or she is in relation to the chair.

SITTING DOWN

STEP 1 When guiding a resident to sit down, guide the resident to a chair.

STEP 2 Describe the chair, for example, if it has arms or rollers.

STEP 3 Tell the resident where he or she is in relation to the chair (in front of the chair, behind the chair).

STEP 4 Place the resident's hand on the back of the chair.

STEP 5 Ask the resident to feel the seat with the other arm, then tell the resident to turn around and sit down.

When helping a resident get into a car, you need to show the resident where the door is and make sure the resident does not bump his or her head while getting in.

GETTING INTO A CAR

STEP 1 When helping a person who is visually impaired to get in a car, guide one hand to the door handle and one hand to the top of the car. Ask the resident to open the door (or open it for the resident) while keeping the other hand on the roof of the car to protect the resident's head.

STEP 2 You may need to support the resident by holding the resident's arm as he or she steps into the car and sits down.

Guiding Someone with Adaptive Equipment

Some residents with visual impairments require adaptive equipment such as a wheelchair, walker, or support cane to walk. Helping them get around requires different techniques.

A resident who uses a walker may prefer to be guided physically or just with words.

USING A WALKER

- When guiding a resident who is using a walker, talk to the resident. Ask if she wants to walk independently while you describe the environment.
- Alternatively, if the resident is hesitant to use the walker independently, place your hand on one of the resident's hands and walk beside the walker as the resident moves. Continue to describe the environment as you walk.
- If you are walking into the sun or in an area with a great deal of glare, the resident's vision may be very blurred. Be prepared to assist if the resident is unable to see to move forward by using sighted guide or getting a wheelchair.

When guiding residents who use a cane for support, remember that they won't be able to grasp your arm with the hand that holds the cane.

USING A SUPPORT CANE

STEP 1 When guiding a resident who is using a support cane, walk on the side away from the cane. The resident may hold onto your forearm if he or she needs more support. Use sighted guide if appropriate.

STEP 2 Continue to describe the environment as you walk. If you are walking into the sun or in an area with a great deal of glare, the resident's vision may be very blurred. Be prepared to assist by offering sighted guide.

Visually impaired residents who use wheelchairs also need to be guided.

USING A WHEELCHAIR

STEP 1 When guiding a resident who is in a wheelchair, talk to the resident and ask if he or she wants to be pushed.

STEP 2 If the resident wants to push himself or herself, you can provide guidance by putting your hand on one of the resident's shoulders.

STEP 3 Describe the environment as you walk. Alert the resident to obstacles in the way.

Self-Protective Techniques

Self-protective techniques are techniques that residents who are visually impaired can use to protect themselves from obstacles when walking alone, without a sighted guide. You can teach these techniques to assist a resident in walking safely alone, in his or her room, or in unfamiliar surroundings.

UPPER-ARM AND FOREARM TECHNIQUE

The upper-arm and forearm technique is designed to protect the resident's upper body and head from obstacles such as open cabinet doors and partially closed doors. Use the following steps to teach this technique to a resident.

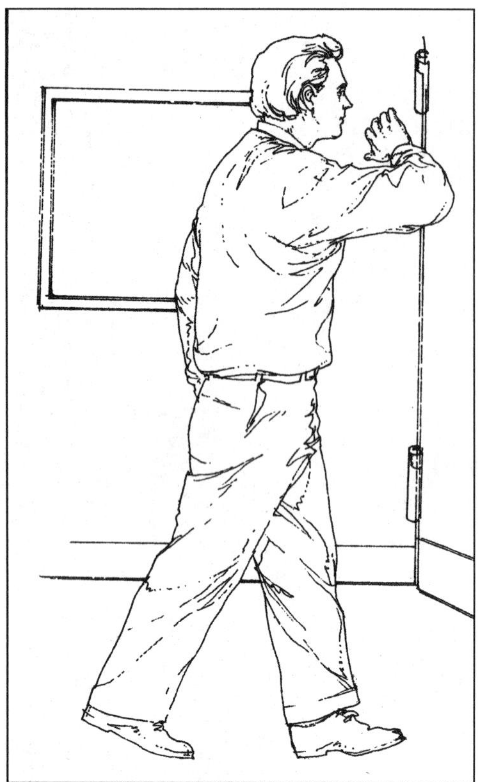

The upper-arm and forearm technique is used to protect the upper body and head against objects a resident might encounter while moving about.

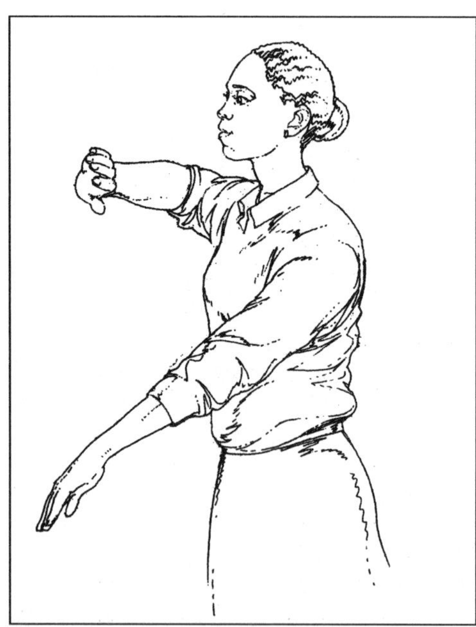

The lower-arm and forearm technique is used to protect the lower body against objects a resident might encounter while moving about.

UPPER-ARM AND FOREARM TECHNIQUE

STEP 1 Tell the resident to use the stronger arm and to extend it forward.

STEP 2 Tell the resident to bend the arm and bring it across the body to the opposite shoulder.

STEP 3 Tell the resident to hold the arm about 8 to 10 inches from the body with the palm outward.

STEP 4 Have the resident lift the arm to place it in front of the face and curl the fingers. This will protect the fingers should the resident run into an object.

STEP 5 Ask the resident to relax while walking.

LOWER-ARM AND FOREARM TECHNIQUE

The lower-arm and forearm technique is designed to protect the lower body when moving about in an area where there may be obstacles. Use the following steps to teach this technique to a resident.

LOWER-ARM AND FOREARM TECHNIQUE

STEP 1 Tell the resident to extend the arm across the lower body at the belly button.

STEP 2 Ask the resident to extend the arm away from the body about 8 to 10 inches.

STEP 3 Ask the resident to curl the fingers and use the back of the hand for protection.

Residents should use the upper-arm and forearm and lower-arm and forearm techniques together for more protection when moving about.

Trailing

Trailing is another way to get around the environment safely by moving the back of the hand along a wall as one moves. It helps a resident keep track of where he or she is while walking through the facility and find specific objects, such as a door. Trailing is commonly done along the right-hand wall. Residents can use this technique to walk independently to specific places in the facility—for example, from their room to the dining room or common room. Use the following steps to teach trailing to a resident.

TRAILING

STEP 1 Tell the resident to stand parallel to a wall and close to it.

STEP 2 Tell the resident to touch the wall with the hand nearest to the wall.

STEP 3 Ask the resident to cup the hand slightly and use the back of the hand to trail along the wall to protect the fingers.

STEP 4 When coming to a doorway, the resident should trail across the doorway leaving the hand in the trailing position and resume on the other side. It is best to use the upper-arm and forearm self-protective technique when trailing across a door to protect the resident from any objects that may protrude from the room.

Learning this technique may take some practice and may require some encouragement and support on your part.

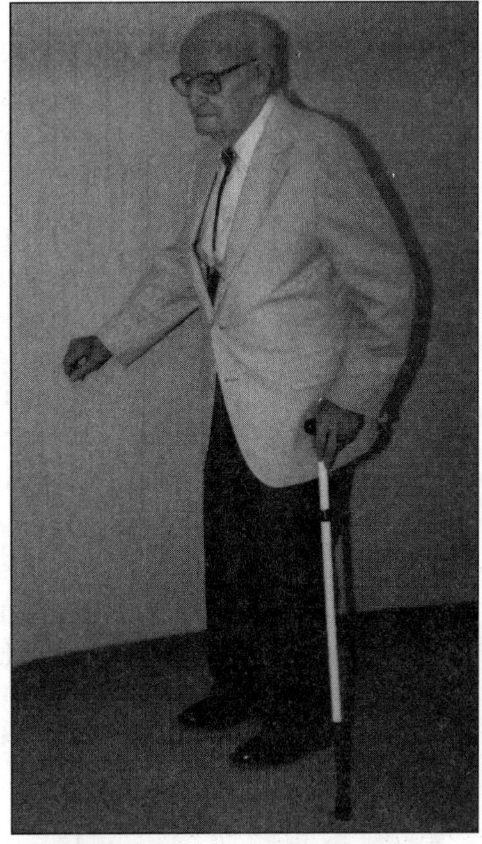

ANN G. HUBBARD

Trailing along a wall helps a resident recognize where he or she is and find specific objects, such as a door.

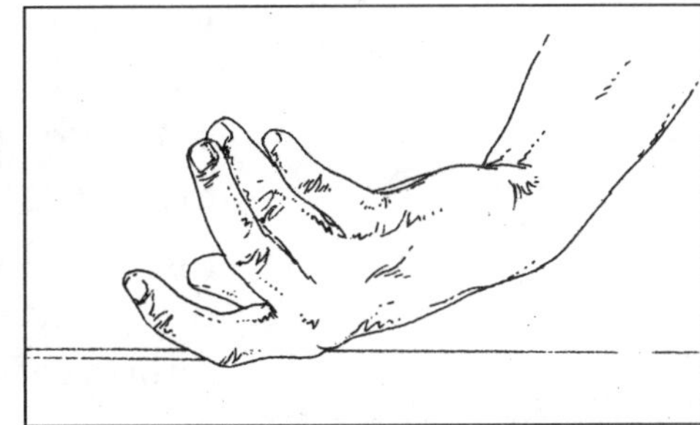

Position of the hand and fingers in trailing.

Orienting the Resident to the Environment

In order for residents who are visually impaired to be able to move around the facility, they have to become familiar with the different rooms and areas, since they cannot see them clearly. They also need to know where the objects are in each room so that they can find them or avoid bumping into them.

ROOM FAMILIARIZATION

You can use one or more techniques to help an older resident with a visual impairment become familiar with his or her room and other parts of the facility. Techniques include the clock method, labeling, the map method, and trailing.

USING THE CLOCK METHOD

Most people are familiar with the face of a clock and can picture where objects are using the clock as a reference. For example, if the resident visualizes standing at 12 o'clock, using the door to the room as a reference point, the resident may be able to visualize the bed at 3 o'clock, the TV at 6 o'clock, the chair at 9 o'clock, and so on.

USING LABELING

Another technique is to teach the resident to assign labels to different walls of a room. The wall with the bed headboard could be the bed wall, another wall could be the closet wall. The resident could tape-record how he or she has labeled the room to help make the layout easy to remember.

If the resident's compass directions are good, labeling walls the north wall, south wall, and so on is also a good technique.

USING THE MAP METHOD

Magnetic boards are available through catalogs listed in Appendix B, and may be used to make a map of the room or facility.

USING THE TRAILING METHOD

Using trailing and self-protective techniques, the resident can practice learning and remembering where objects are located in the room or in other parts of the facility.

HAZARDS AND OBSTACLES

Encourage residents who are visually impaired to be as independent as possible. This means making sure that both the residents and the staff do their part to ensure safety. The resident may use memorization and other methods to remember where objects are placed. If objects in the resident's environment are moved without the resident's knowledge, they may become obstacles. It is also important to be aware of potential hazards in the environment—such as area rugs that can slide underfoot, doors left ajar that a resident might walk into, and raised door thresholds that a resident might trip over—and guard against them.

The following guidelines will help you prevent hazards for visually impaired residents who are moving around in the facility.

PREVENTING HAZARDS IN THE ENVIRONMENT

- Never move furniture in the resident's room or immediate environment without telling and reminding the resident.
- Area rugs are dangerous because they can slide underfoot; they should not be used if they cannot be secured.

- Remember to close doors and not leave them open partway.
- Thresholds should be installed to be as flush to the floor as possible. Work with residents to ensure they are aware of thresholds in the facility that might pose a hazard. Painting thresholds a contrasting color may help some residents who can see color.
- Residents who are visually impaired and who do not use canes should be encouraged to use self-protective techniques when venturing outside their room.

NAVIGATING HALLWAYS

Hallways can be disorienting for a resident and in order to navigate them safely, residents should be aware of some techniques that can help them to be oriented.

- Trailing (to move one's fingers along a wall using the back of the hand) is one technique for navigating hallways safely.
- Eliminate glare in hallways.
- Use effective contrast in wall coverings.
- Use appropriate signs, such as large-print and high-contrast signs that contrast with the walls to identify rooms and exits. High contrast makes it easier to read (see Appendix C, Tips for Print Readability).
- Ensure signs are properly illuminated and well marked, with signage at eye level.
- Eliminate potential hazards such as protruding furniture or objects, use of high-gloss waxes, and equipment or other items lying in the halls.

LOCATING THE PARTS OF THE FACILITY

You should orient the resident with a visual impairment to the location of the different rooms in the facility, such as the dining room. This is easy to do by encouraging the use of the trailing technique as you guide the resident through the facility and point out specific clues, such as smells and sounds, that identify each area. For example, the smell of food and rattling of dishes are clues that you are near the dining room. You can also use specific directions to a particular room (for example, "Turn right at the elevators to get to the TV room"). Also, a tactile map (a map that has raised lines) of the facility is useful in helping residents who are visually impaired become oriented to the facility.

FINDING THE RESIDENT'S ROOM

The resident may wish to "mark" his or her room to make it easier to find. The room can be identified by using a visual or tactile cue, such as a rubber band or a ribbon on the doorknob or a decal on the door or on a railing near the door.

To make it easier to find the key to the room, the resident can use a particular-colored key for the room or mark the key with a piece of tape, a raised dot, or special key ring to differentiate that key from others. By feeling the edge of the key, the resident can tell which way to insert the key to open the door. Plastic keys can also be marked to indicate which side is right side up by placing a sticker on the top or punching a hole in the upper right corner.

USING AN ELEVATOR

Elevator signs should be in large print and at eye level. If the resident has difficulty knowing on which floor to get off, try placing some tape or another mark that the resident can feel (tactile marking) just outside the elevator door of the resident's floor.

Congratulations! You have reached the end of Lesson 5. Now go on to the Key Points to review what you have learned in this lesson.

KEY POINTS IN LESSON 5

Getting Around the Environment

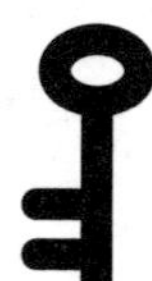

1. The three important techniques to teach residents who are visually impaired for getting around in their environment are
   - sighted guide for walking with the resident
   - self-protective techniques
   - trailing
2. Important points to remember about orienting the resident to the environment are how to
   - orient the resident to his or her room
   - prevent hazards in the environment
   - help the resident to find his or her room
   - help the resident to find other areas in the facility

LEARNING ACTIVITIES

Try the following activities to practice what you have learned in this lesson. Some of the activities involve the use of simulators—glasses that simulate different types of vision loss. (See Appendix B for sources of vision simulators.) It is important to work in pairs while doing these exercises. One person uses the simulators while the other watches for safety and provides feedback.

- Using the simulators with another staff member, take turns practicing sighted guide techniques such as walking around the facility, opening and going through doors, and sitting.
- Try the sighted guide technique with a resident who uses a walker and with another resident who uses a wheelchair.
- Using the simulators, practice the upper-arm and forearm technique in a kitchen area where you have left cabinet doors open.
- Using the simulators, try trailing from a resident's room to the dining hall.
- Using the simulators, try opening a door with a key.

SELF-CHECK

Indicate whether each statement is true (T) or false (F) in the space provided. Check Appendix A for the answers. Then go back and review any statements you may have missed.

______ 1. When walking with a resident who is visually impaired, I should hold on to the person tightly and push the resident in front of me.

______ 2. When helping a resident who is visually impaired to take a seat, I should try to pick up and place the resident in the chair.

______ 3. Self-protective techniques can protect the upper body and the lower body.

PART 2 SPECIAL SKILL AREAS

LESSON 6 Maintaining Personal Hygiene

GOALS

- ➤ To know the areas of personal hygiene with which a resident who is visually impaired may have trouble.
- ➤ To know the types of assistance that may be most helpful.

OBJECTIVE

At the end of this lesson, you will be able to assist the resident with learning bathing and grooming techniques to enhance independence.

TEACH Principles

When working with a resident who is visually impaired to help him or her with personal hygiene, use the five TEACH principles:

T—**Talk** to the resident about what you are teaching him or her to do.

E—**Encourage** the resident to try the techniques in this lesson.

- **A—Assess** the resident's ability to get around safely in the bathroom and to accomplish grooming tasks.
- **C—"Can do"** is the motto for each resident.
- **H—Help** the resident to make needed changes in the bathroom and learn the techniques he or she wishes to use for grooming.

Assisting Residents with Bathing

Bathing is an important area of personal hygiene for all residents. It affects the resident's self-esteem as well as health. Even a slight degree of vision loss, however, can make it difficult for a resident who is visually impaired to function independently in the bathroom. Some of the problems that often occur in the bathroom are

- poor lighting
- presence of glare
- lack of contrast
- potential hazards such as area rugs

KEY SOLUTIONS IN THE BATHROOM

To find solutions to some of the problems that tend to occur in the bathroom, remember the key solutions discussed in Lesson 1. Solutions that will help with bathing include

- increasing lighting
- eliminating glare
- eliminating hazards
- using color contrast
- labeling items
- organizing items

For more information about functional environments in general, see Appendix E, Creating a Functional Environment for Older People Who Are Visually Impaired.

SUFFICIENT AND APPROPRIATE LIGHTING

Often, bathrooms lack enough lighting over the tub or shower area. Additional lighting can be helpful for all older residents. Compact fluorescent bulbs or full-spectrum bulbs such as Chromalux bulbs discussed in Lesson 4 may help to eliminate glare and emit sufficient light. An adjustable swing-arm lamp might add light to the mirror area for applying makeup and combing hair.

NONSKID RUGS

Replace area rugs with nonskid rugs in a color that contrasts with the floor. The use of a contrasting color will make it much easier for a resident who is visually impaired to see the rug; getting around the bathroom will therefore become easier and safer.

CONTRAST

Use of contrast is one of the key solutions discussed in Lesson 1. It is one of the most effective methods for helping residents with visual impairments get around in the environment.

Place a contrasting-color nonskid mat, friction tape, or patterned appliqués on the bottom of the tub or the floor of the shower to prevent falls. The use of contrasting tape also helps residents judge depth more accurately.

If grab bars are used in the shower or tub area, covering them with brightly colored tape will improve contrast with the walls and make them much more visible to the resident.

Use towels, washcloths, and bath mats that contrast in color with the tub, the tile, and also the walls. Use of contrasting, darker colors will make the towels easier to see and reduce glare in the bathroom.

It is easier to find a wall light switch or a bathroom cup if the object contrasts in color with the walls. A white toilet seat can be replaced with a colored one to increase contrast.

ORGANIZATION AND LABELING

Organization and labeling are two other key solutions to helping the resident to function independently. Keep frequently used items such as soap, shampoo, and conditioner in the same place at all times so that the resident can find and identify them more easily. Using a shower caddy of contrasting color is a good way to organize these items.

It is easier to identify items when they are shaped differently than when the containers are the same. When possible, use plastic containers rather than glass to prevent breakage. It is easy to label or mark these kinds of items with a strip of colored tape or a rubber band. For example, use a strip of colored or black tape on the shampoo and no tape on the conditioner.

TECHNIQUES FOR BATHING

REGULATING WATER TEMPERATURE

You can teach the resident how to regulate the temperature of the bathwater by teaching him or her how far to turn the handle to get the desired temperature. Contrasting-color tape can be placed on the hot or cold handle to help the resident identify which is hot and which is cold.

A single-knob faucet can be marked to indicate a comfortable water setting by using a piece of tape or raised marker.

To prevent burns when filling a tub, always turn on cold water first, then add hot. Turn off the hot water first, then the cold.

FILLING THE BATHTUB

Sometimes it is difficult for a resident with a visual impairment to tell the depth of the water in the tub. Putting a contrasting stripe of tape at the desired depth of water in the tub or draping a contrasting-color bath mat or towel over the tub helps the resident judge the depth of the water. A floating object, such as a child's rubber duck or other small colored bath toy, can also be used to indicate the water levels in the bathtub and sink.

Grooming Techniques

Maintaining their appearance can be important for the morale and self-esteem of residents, as well as for their health. Residents with visual impairments often need help to find new methods of accomplishing grooming tasks that once were routine.

BRUSHING TEETH

You may need to teach the resident how to locate and apply toothpaste to toothbrush independently. The following are some helpful hints for tooth brushing:

- Use a dark-colored toothpaste or striped toothpaste to contrast with white toothbrush bristles. White toothpaste with dark bristles will work equally well.
- The resident should hold the bristles of the brush between the thumb and forefinger. This way the resident can squeeze the toothpaste onto the brush.
- The resident can also squeeze the toothpaste onto a forefinger and then put it on the brush.
- Squeeze a small amount of toothpaste into the palm of the hand and then scoop up the toothpaste onto the bristles of the toothbrush.
- If the resident is the only one using the paste, he or she may prefer to squeeze the paste directly into the mouth.

HAIR CARE

It is often difficult for a resident who is visually impaired to see if his or her hair is combed or brushed the way he or she wants it to be. The following are some useful hints to help residents fix their own hair:

- Use a magnifying mirror to enlarge the face and head area.
- Drape a contrasting towel around the resident's shoulders to make the head and hair more visible.
- Alternatively, install a high towel bar across from the mirror in the bathroom and hang a contrasting towel on it to provide contrast to the resident's view of his or her hair in the mirror.

SHAVING

An electric shaver is a safer option for a resident who is visually impaired. However, some residents may insist on using a manual razor. Some useful hints are as follows:

- Use a magnifying mirror to enlarge the face and head area.
- Applying shaving cream to one area of the face at a time may also provide enough contrast to allow the resident to identify the area of the face that needs to be shaved. The shaving cream also provides a different texture, so the resident can tell where to shave by touching his face.

NAIL CARE

Nail care is often difficult for a resident with visual impairment to accomplish. Some helpful hints are as follows:

- Short nails are easier to maintain.
- Nails should be cleaned with a nail brush and soap and water.
- For many older people, especially those who are visually impaired, using a nail file is an easier and safer way to care for nails than cutting them.
- A nail block—a four-sided nail file—is sometimes easier for an older person to hold and manipulate.

Residents with diabetes who are visually impaired need to be especially careful with nail care. They should avoid cutting their nails at all, especially the toenails, because if they accidently cut themselves, healing may be difficult—and a visually impaired person may not notice that a cut needs medical attention.

APPLYING MAKEUP

Applying makeup may be tedious for some residents with low vision, but it can be mastered with practice if it is important to the resident. A lighted magnifying mirror may help the resident to see what she is doing.

Teaching a resident to use a systematic approach can help her to be more independent in putting on her makeup. The following suggestions can help:

- Labeling. First label the cosmetics, using the techniques discussed in Lesson 1.
- Use facial landmarks. Identify and use facial landmarks to determine where to apply cosmetics such as eye shadow or blush. For example:
  - The edge of the eyebrow is a good landmark to use in deciding how far out toward the side of the face eye shadow should go.
  - The bottom of the nose or the base of the cheekbone can form a boundary for applying blush.
- Use counting techniques. It can be helpful for the resident to count the number of drops of foundation needed for sufficient coverage, such as one drop on each cheek, the nose, the chin, and the forehead. She can also count the number of brush strokes needed to apply the right amount of blush or eye shadow.
- Another way to apply foundation is to apply a thin line of foundation down the center of the face, using fingers to blend up and out. Using fingers in place of brushes or sponges can help with control of the amount of color and accurate placement of the cosmetics on the face.
- Use powder instead of creams. Powdered foundation may be easier to use than creams because it allows the user more control over the amount of color used.
- Use subtle shades. Using subtle shades of cosmetics may make uneven or inconsistent application less noticeable and decrease the visibility of any errors.
- Get feedback. The resident needs to get feedback from a sighted person to determine if this systematic approach to applying makeup is working.

Congratulations! You have finished Lesson 6. Now go on to the Key Points to review what you have learned in this lesson.

KEY POINTS IN LESSON 6

Maintaining Personal Hygiene

1. Some of the problems a resident may confront in the bathroom are
   - ➤ lack of good lighting
   - ➤ glare
   - ➤ lack of contrast
   - ➤ potential hazards, such as area rugs with no backing
2. Some solutions for these problems include
   - ➤ increasing lighting
   - ➤ eliminating glare
   - ➤ eliminating hazards
   - ➤ using color contrast
   - ➤ labeling items
   - ➤ organizing items in the bath

LEARNING ACTIVITIES

Try the following activities to practice what you have learned in this lesson. Some of the activities involve the use of simulators—glasses that simulate different types of vision loss. (See Appendix B for sources of vision simulators.) It is important to work in pairs while doing these exercises. One person uses the simulators while the other watches for safety and provides feedback.

Using the simulators, try brushing your teeth.

Using the simulators, try filling a white tub with water.

In a bathroom lit by a single 60-watt bulb, try seeing your face in the mirror and applying lipstick.

☑ SELF-CHECK

Indicate whether each statement is true (T) or false (F) in the space provided. Check Appendix A for the answers. Then go back and review any statements you may have missed.

______ 1. Effective lighting is essential to safety in the bathroom.

______ 2. Transferring toothpaste to a toothbrush can be made easier by teaching the resident to first apply the paste to a finger and then to the brush.

______ 3. Dark towels and a dark bath mat provide the most contrast against white walls and flooring.

______ 4. Reducing glare is critical in the bathroom.

LESSON 7 Managing Medications

GOAL

To learn various methods of identifying and self-administering medication independently and safely.

OBJECTIVE

At the end of the lesson, you will be able to suggest methods for managing medication safely.

TEACH Principles

When helping a resident who is visually impaired to manage medications, use the five TEACH principles.

T—**Talk** to the resident about what you are teaching him or her to do.

E—**Encourage** the resident to try the techniques in this lesson.

A—**Assess** the resident's ability to take medications safely and correctly.

- **C—"Can do"** is the motto for each resident.
- **H—Help** the resident to organize medications for easy identification if he or she wishes to do so.

Medication Safety

Older people typically take more than one medication. Some residents may be able to manage their own medications. For self-administering of medication to be possible, residents must be able to identify each medication they take.

Being able to identify each medication is extremely important. Inability to read pill bottles can lead to mistakes with serious consequences. It is especially important, therefore, for older people who are visually impaired to develop a system that allows easy and safe identification of medications.

To start, it is always possible to ask the pharmacist to print a large-print label for the pill bottle. If this isn't large enough for the resident to see, you can help the resident to use other visual and tactile labels and systems of organization.

Organizing Medications

Use a dark-colored tray when organizing a resident's medications. The tray can provide contrast with the medication containers to help with identifying them. A tray also has a raised edge that can catch pills if they are dropped and prevent them from rolling onto the floor.

The size and shape of a pill can help with identification. The resident can practice feeling the different shapes and sizes of the pills.

Labeling Medications

The ability to label personal items is an important skill for a resident to acquire in order to continue to function independently. You can help set up a system for the resident's medications.

Different sizes and even colors of rubber bands can be used to differentiate between medicine bottles. Also, strips of tape can be used in different directions—vertical, horizontal, or zigzag. When attaching labels to medication bottles, be sure to place them on the side of the bottle that does not have the label so that someone else can still help the resident by reading the print.

Medication bottles can also be distinguished by size and shape. Most bottles are the same color, however. Another method of organization is to keep medicines in alphabetical order.

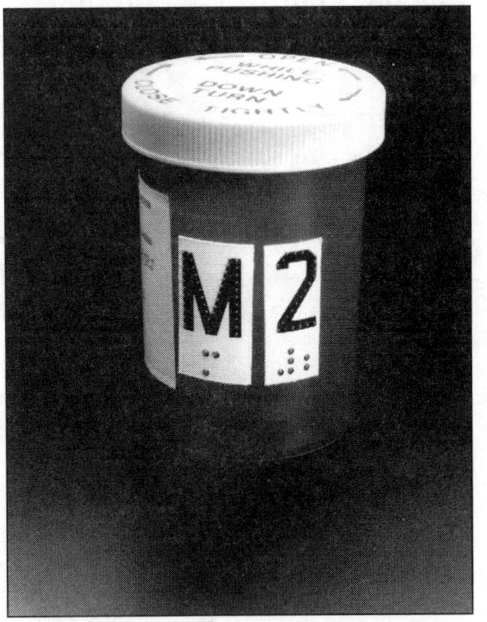

ROBERT HAKALSKI/VISUAL MACHINERY

This medicine container is labeled with a combination of large print, tactile markings (dots along the letters), and braille letters.

Using Pill Boxes

Weekly pill boxes—these are plastic boxes with a section for every day of the week—are often useful to residents who are visually impaired. You can help sort the medications into the sections of the box, and the resident can self- administer them.

Some prescription bottles come with an alarm system to remind the resident when to take medications (these can be ordered from the catalogs listed in Appendix B).

Talking Prescription Labels

Several systems are available that can identify medications and give information about them by speaking aloud the information written on the labels. See the Resources in Appendix B for more details.

Magnifying Prescription Labels

Products that enlarge the prescription label, such as the Medifier, are available through the catalogs listed in Appendix B. The magnifier fits all standard prescription vials.

Congratulations! You have reached the end of Lesson 7. Now go on to the Key Points to review what you have learned in this lesson.

KEY POINTS IN LESSON 7

Managing Medications

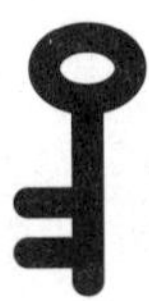

1. There are several techniques for labeling medications, such as using large print, tactile labels, and color coding.
2. Organizing medications in order to differentiate among them is critical for safety.

LEARNING ACTIVITIES

Try the following activities to practice what you have learned in this lesson. Some of the activities involve the use of vision simulators—glasses that simulate different types of vision loss. (See Appendix B for sources of vision simulators.) It is important to work in pairs while doing these exercises. One person uses the simulators while the other watches for safety and provides feedback.

Using simulators, try identifying large-print labels on pill bottles.

Organize pill bottles using a system you have designed. Using simulators, try to identify the bottles on a different day. Or, ask another staff member to organize the pill bottles for you—using a method you have chosen—and then try to identify them.

SELF-CHECK

Indicate whether each statement is true (T) or false (F) in the space provided. Check Appendix A for the answers. Then go back and review any statements you may have missed.

______ 1. Helping the resident devise a labeling system for medicine bottles is critical.

______ 2. Talking medicine bottles are available commercially.

LESSON 8 Eating Techniques

GOAL

To enable you to instruct the resident with a visual impairment to eat as independently as possible.

OBJECTIVE

At the end of the session you will be able to demonstrate to an older resident with a visual impairment how to locate foods and beverages at a place setting and to eat independently and efficiently.

Teach Principles

When working with a resident who is visually impaired to help him or her with eating techniques, use the five TEACH principles.

T—**Talk** to the resident about problems she may have with eating.

E—**Encourage** the resident to try the techniques in this lesson.

- **A—Assess** the resident and the dining environment.
- **C—"Can do"** is the motto for each resident.
- **H—Help** the resident to become independent in eating.

Solutions for Eating Independently

Mealtime can be difficult for residents who are visually impaired. They may not know what food is on the plate or be able to find the food they want to eat. They may accidentally spill food or beverages. You can teach residents techniques that will help them eat more independently.

As discussed in Lesson 3, contrast is a useful technique to help some residents with visual impairments to distinguish objects, including the dishes on the table. Using the clock method is helpful in describing to the resident the location of food on a plate. An alternative method is using compass directions. These methods are explained in more detail later in this lesson. Foods can sometimes also be identified by aroma and temperature.

To avoid glare that can make it even harder to see what is on the table, a visually impaired resident should be seated with his or her back to a window. The quantity and quality of lighting in the dining room should also be considered to eliminate glare.

Adaptive equipment that can help with eating can be ordered from the catalogs listed in Appendix B. These items include

- plate guards or food bumpers
- rocker knives
- adapted utensils
- scoop dishes
- plates with raised rims
- liquid level indicator

Use of Contrast in Preparing the Place Setting

As explained, the use of contrast is helpful to many persons with visual impairments. Work with the dining room staff to make use of contrasting colors in place settings to make it easier for residents to see them. For example, use a dark tablecloth with white dishes. (Generally, dark on light is easiest to see.) Solid colors are better than patterns.

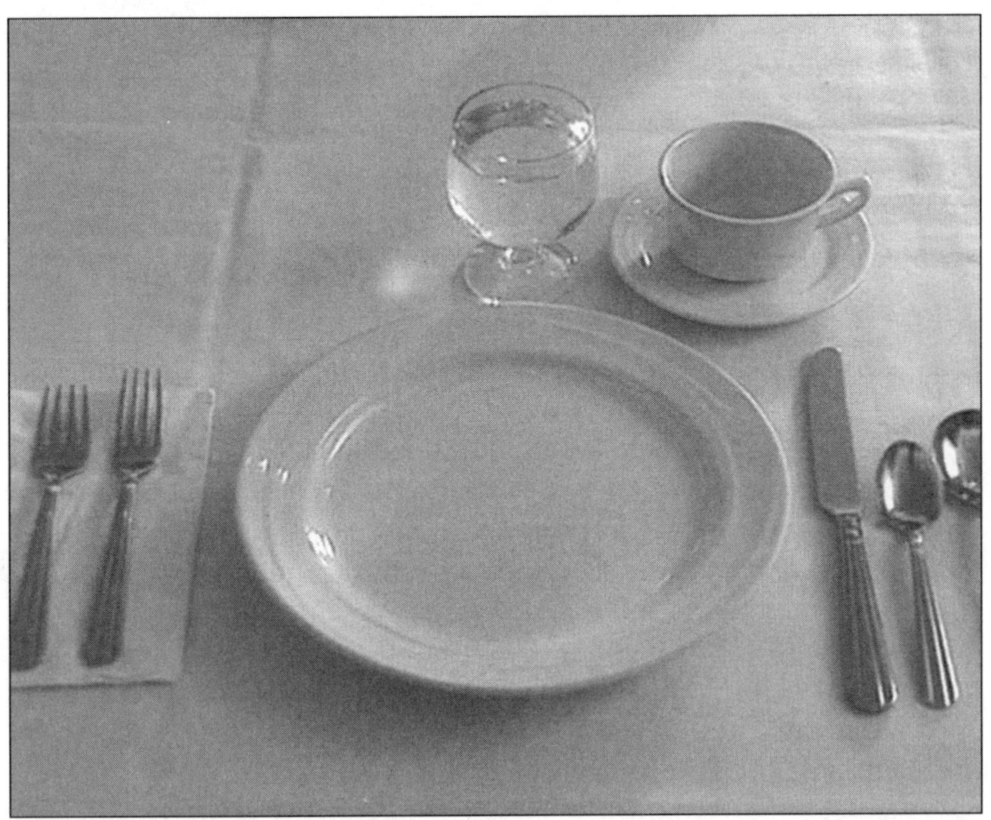

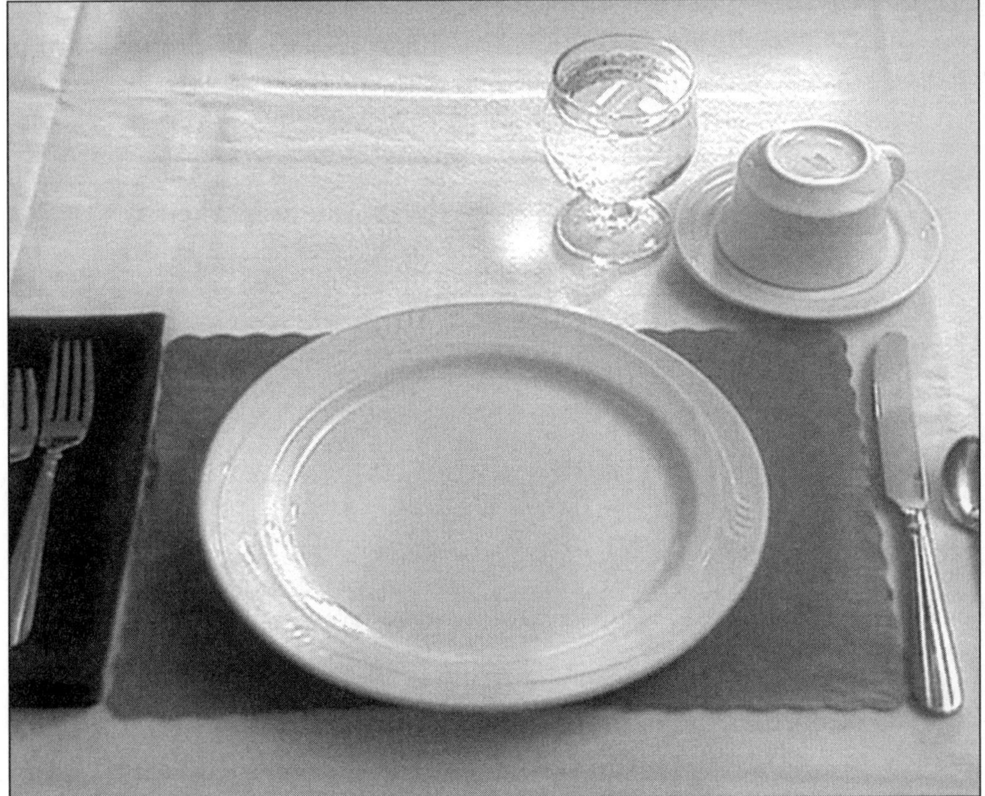

AMERICAN FOUNDATION FOR THE BLIND

The white dishes and clear glass seem to blend into the white tablecloth. Using a placemat and napkin of a contrasting color makes the place setting easier to see.

Clear glasses should never be used for clear liquids since it is difficult for a person with a visual impairment to detect the liquid. Coffee should be placed in a white or light-colored cup or mug. It may be helpful to use a tray of a contrasting color to keep the place setting in a confined area.

Methods for Locating Items on the Table

You can teach residents to locate the items in their place setting and the food on their plate. It is helpful to think of the place setting or the plate as the face of a clock. Then you can tell the resident what is located at various numbers on the "clock." Alternatively, you can use compass directions to tell the resident where items are located (for example, at due north, or in the southwest section of the plate) instead of the clock method. The principle is the same.

To teach a resident how to find items in the place setting and on the plate, use the following steps:

STEP 1 Describe place setting. Describe to the resident the layout of the place setting. For example, explain where the coffee cup is (usually at 1:00 o'clock), the water glass (at 12 o'clock), the napkin (at

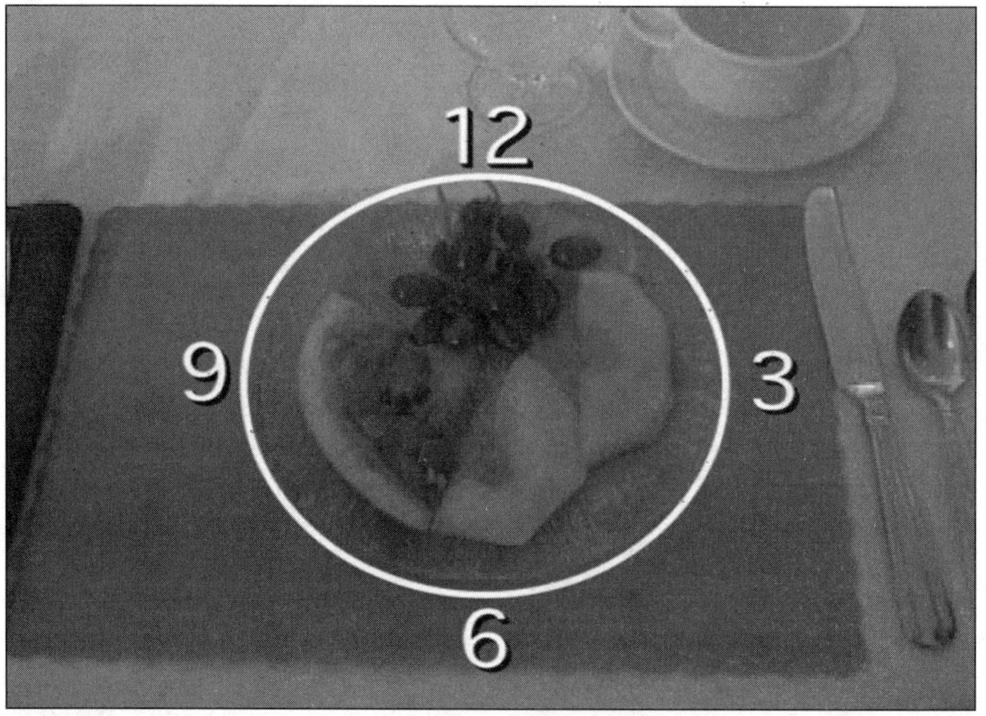

AMERICAN FOUNDATION FOR THE BLIND

A good way to describe the location of food on a plate is to pretend the plate is a clock face and explain which number the food is near.

9 o'clock), the plate (at 6:00 o'clock), the salt and pepper shakers (at 2 o'clock), and so forth.

STEP 2 Describe food on the plate. Repeat the clock method technique to tell the resident where food items are on the plate (for example, grapes at 12 o'clock and melon at 3 o'clock).

STEP 3 Use location techniques. Explain to the resident how to locate objects without knocking over glasses and other tall items by trailing the hand along the tabletop. This is accomplished by holding the back of the hand against the table and moving gently around the place setting to locate glasses and cups. It is helpful to always use the same pattern for the table setting so that the resident knows where to look for the glasses and cups.

STEP 4 Memorize where items are. To help the resident memorize where items are in the place setting, once the resident has located an item, such as a coffee cup, have the resident lift the cup and place it back in the original spot. This movement helps to commit the location to memory.

Techniques for Eating

Once the resident is able to locate beverages, utensils, and the items on the plate, he or she can learn a number of techniques that will help the resident with the food, including how to spread with a knife, how to cut with a knife, ways to eat gracefully, and pouring hot and cold liquids.

SPREADING FOOD USING A TABLE KNIFE

STEP 1 Locate cutting edge of knife. Help the resident find the cutting edge of the knife with his or her fingers.

STEP 2 Locate spread(s). Tell the resident where to locate the spread (butter, jam, mayonnaise) using the clock method.

STEP 3 Determine amount of butter, for example. If the resident is spreading butter, ask the resident to run the knife over the butter dish to determine how much butter there is and how much is needed for the bread or other food.

STEP 4 Cut a portion. You should instruct the resident to cut off the desired portion of butter and place it in the center of the bread. From there the resident can spread it to the edges, using the fingers as a guide to the edges.

CUTTING FOODS USING A KNIFE

This section explains how to cut with a regular knife; however, using a rocker knife (available from the catalogs listed in Appendix B), which has a vertical handle and cuts with a downward push and a side-to-side rocking action, may be easier for some residents. Residents may need assistance with this task.

STEP 1 Find cutting edge of knife. Ask the resident to find the cutting edge of the knife with the fingers and to hold the knife with the blade facing down. An alternative method is to drag the edge of the knife on the edge of the plate and listen or feel for serrations.

STEP 2 Tell the resident to locate the edge of the meat he or she wants to cut by putting the knife on the edge of the meat.

STEP 3 Then tell the resident to put the fork into the meat about a half-inch, or the width of a mouthful, from the edge.

STEP 4 Cut a portion. Instruct the resident to cut in a semicircle around the fork with the knife. The resident can tell when the meat is cut through by pressing the fork into and under the food and pulling; the resident will feel a "drag" if the piece of meat has not been fully cut.

STEP 5 Cut remainder into portions. The resident can then cut the entire piece of meat in the same fashion, always using the knife to maintain contact with the meat.

When cutting meat and vegetables, placing a non-slippery mat under the plate may anchor the plate and keep it from moving.

EATING GRACEFULLY

- A piece of bread or a knife can be used as a buffer to push the food onto the fork.
- Anchoring the plate by using a nonskid mat under it and using a plate guard or plate with raised rim will reduce spillage.
- Spillage can be reduced if the resident's body is properly aligned with the place setting and the resident's head and face are positioned over the plate.
- Using a napkin in the resident's lap, and tucking it in if possible, will protect clothing.

POURING COLD LIQUIDS

Using contrast will help most residents when they are trying to pour liquids. For example, use a white pitcher for dark liquids such as iced tea. Teach residents the following steps for pouring liquids.

STEP 1 Locate the pitcher. Ask the resident to trail along the table with the dominant hand to locate the pitcher.

STEP 2 Locate the spout. Have the resident locate the spout by moving the hand up the pitcher. Then turn the pitcher until the spout faces the glass.

STEP 3 Move the glass. Instruct the resident to move the glass toward the pitcher, using the index finger on the spout of the pitcher.

STEP 4 Raise the glass. Have the resident raise the glass with the other hand, wrapping the middle finger and thumb around the glass and placing the index finger over the top edge into the glass.

STEP 5 Lift the pitcher. The resident can then lift the pitcher slightly and touch the spout of the pitcher to the rim of the glass. The resident should lift the glass slightly to feel the weight change in the glass while pouring.

STEP 6 Pour. The resident can then pour until he or she can feel the water or other liquid reach the index finger. The resident should also listen for sound changes as liquid reaches the top of the glass.

Alternative technique: Residents may prefer to use a device called an electronic liquid-level indicator—also known as "say when"—to determine when the liquid reaches the top of the cup or glass. The liquid-level indicator is placed over the lip of a cup. The same technique for pouring can be used, except that the resident does not put his or her finger on the cup. The device is battery operated and beeps when the liquid reaches the top. These devices are available from the catalogs listed in Appendix B.

Work with the resident to practice these techniques outside mealtimes to avoid embarrassment and to lessen frustration for the resident. It may be easier to practice with empty containers first and to pour over a tray to catch any spills.

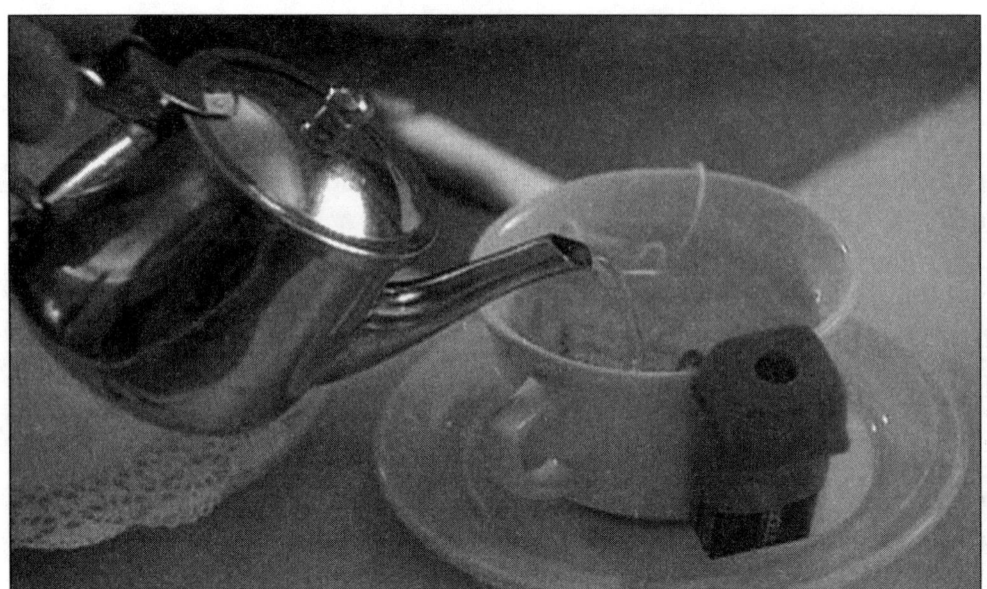

AMERICAN FOUNDATION FOR THE BLIND

A liquid-level indicator beeps when liquid gets near the top of the cup.

POURING HOT LIQUIDS

Pouring hot liquids can be dangerous, especially for an older person and especially for a resident with neuropathy, loss of sensitivity in the fingertips. It is safer for a resident to use an electronic liquid-level indicator for pouring hot liquids. Residents may need assistance with this task.

IDENTIFYING CONDIMENTS

Teach the resident to use the following cues to identify condiments or seasonings such as salt, pepper, ketchup, and mustard:

- weight
- aroma
- sound
- color
- size of holes in shaker (for example, holes for salt are often larger than those for pepper)

ADDING SALT AND PEPPER

To make sure residents don't add too much salt or pepper to their food, teach them to use the following method:

STEP 1 Instruct the resident to pour a little salt or pepper into the palm of one hand.

STEP 2 The resident can then take a pinch of salt or pepper with the other hand and place it on the food a little at a time. (See Lesson 7, Safe Techniques for Preparing Foods).

Congratulations! You have reached the end of Lesson 8. Now go on to the Key Points to review what you have learned in this lesson.

KEY POINTS IN LESSON 8

Eating Techniques

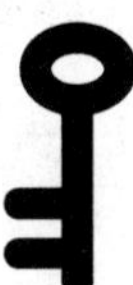

1. Contrast, lighting, and glare control are critical principles to remember in setting up the dining environment.
2. The clock method is a useful technique to use in orienting a resident to the table setting, food placement, and other items on the table, such as the salt and pepper shakers.

LEARNING ACTIVITIES

Try the following activities to practice what you have learned in this lesson. Some of the activities involve the use of simulators—glasses that simulate different types of vision loss. (See Appendix B for sources of vision simulators.) It is important to work in pairs while doing these exercises. One person uses the simulators while the other watches for safety and provides feedback.

- Have another staff member set up a place setting for you. Identify where the different items in the place setting are using the clock method.
- Using the simulators, try to find the items at the place setting and on your plate.
- Using the simulators, try cutting some foods, buttering bread, and pouring liquids.
- Try to explain the eating techniques you have learned in this lesson to another staff person.

☑ SELF-CHECK

Indicate whether each statement is true (T) or false (F) in the space provided. Check Appendix A for the answers. Then go back and review any statements you may have missed.

______ 1. At mealtimes, residents who are visually impaired should never be expected to feed themselves.

______ 2. The clock method is a good method to use when describing a table setting to a resident.

______ 3. There are two techniques for pouring cold liquids, but only one technique is really safe for pouring hot liquids.

LESSON 9 Reading Techniques

GOAL

To explain reading options such as large-print and talking books to the resident who is visually impaired.

OBJECTIVE

At the end of the lesson, you will be able to discuss various reading options with the resident.

Teach Principles

When teaching a resident about the different options for reading, use the five TEACH principles for working successfully with a resident who is visually impaired:

T—Talk to the resident about reading.

E—Encourage the resident to try some of the reading options in this lesson.

A—Assess the resident's reading options.

C—"Can do" is the motto for each resident.

- **H—Help** the resident to become more independent in reading.

Options for Reading

Reading is a near-distance task that uses mainly the central portion of one's vision. Therefore, reading is difficult for older people who have a central field loss—a blind spot in the center of their visual field—such as residents with macular degeneration (see Lesson 3, Overview of Vision Loss).

There are different solutions that can help residents with vision loss continue to read. Some involve reading aids—devices that can make reading easier—and others involve alternative types of reading materials.

Reading Aids

There are a number of devices that can help make reading easier for residents with visual impairments, including everyday tools such as lamps, and devices that are best prescribed by an eye care professional, such as magnifiers.

LIGHTING

Making sure there is enough light of the right type is very important to help residents make the best use of their vision to read. To assess the lighting in a particular area, review the information about lighting in Lesson 4 and try the following solutions to increase lighting for reading:

INCREASING THE LIGHTING FOR READING

- *Task lighting*, a lamp or light that can be adjusted to focus the light directly on a near task, can be used such as reading or needlework.
- A swing-arm lamp or gooseneck lamp that can be positioned over the material or activity is excellent for reading and other near tasks.
- Higher-wattage bulbs produce more light, but the manufacturer's recommended wattage for the lamp should not be exceeded.
- White or light-colored lamp shades allow more light to fall on a near task.

- Compact fluorescent lamps (CFLs) for ambient lighting provide good illumination and produce less heat than do lamps with incandescent bulbs. Incandescent bulbs are good for reading, as are combination lamps that feature both fluorescent and incandescent lighting.
- Chromalux bulbs provide full-spectrum lighting for reading.

HAND HELD OR STAND MAGNIFIERS

Residents may benefit by using a handheld magnifier or stand magnification device that is placed directly on the page when reading.

It is much better for the resident if a magnifier is prescribed by a low vision specialist, rather than simply purchased in the stationery store or drugstore. This is because various degrees of magnification work best for different people. A low vision specialist can determine how much magnification is best for each person. Also, when a resident has a low vision examination, the resident can try out various devices at the low vision office. Once a device is chosen, the resident can bring the device back to the residence and test it out in the environment in which it will be used.

You will need to help the resident begin to use the magnifier. The older resident will not automatically be able to use a magnifier successfully without a little instruction, trial and error, and practice. For example, the resident needs to learn at what distance from the printed material the magnifier should be held. You can tell the resident to move the magnifier up and down until the print is in focus. The resident needs to know this is often a difficult task that requires practice and patience.

Using a reading stand to hold the reading material at the best angle and distance can also help some residents keep the material in proper focus.

CLOSED-CIRCUIT TELEVISIONS

A *closed-circuit television* (CCTV) is a reading device that magnifies printed material, which can be very useful for a resident with visual impairment. The CCTV uses a video camera to focus on the material to be viewed. The enlarged image is displayed on a television monitor. A low vision specialist can prescribe the device for a resident with low vision.

There are a variety of CCTVs on the market that are developed and distributed by different companies. Each has special features, so the resident should see several models before making a decision about what is best. The resident may be able to try out a CCTV at the low vision specialist's office. If not, distributors can bring them to the facility to be tested before they are bought.

To use a CCTV, reading materials or other items, such as photographs, are placed on a flat surface. A camera focuses on the printed material and projects an image of the page on a monitor similar to a television screen.

The resident will need to learn how to use the CCTV's controls to move the reading material so that the camera scans from left to right across a line of text and then back to the next line on the left-hand side. It can be a bit frustrating to learn at first, so your support and encouragement can be very helpful. If you are somewhat familiar with how the device operates, you can be very helpful to the resident.

Alternative Reading Materials

Residents who have trouble reading regular print may find it easier to read a book in another format, such as large print, or listen to it on tape.

LARGE-PRINT MATERIALS

Reading materials that are printed in enlarged type can be very helpful for residents who are visually impaired. The technical size for large print is 18 point. Some mainstream periodicals have large-print editions such as *Reader's Digest* and *Newsweek*. The *New York Times* publishes a small weekly edition in large print. There are also publishers that specialize in large-print books, and some large publishing companies have large-print divisions, such as the Doubleday Book Club. (See Appendix B for more information.)

Large-print publications can make reading easier for most older people, many of whom experience some degree of age-related vision loss. They can be very worthwhile purchases for a library in a residential setting. Large-print materials are often available in public libraries as well.

When the facility prints its own items, such as calendars, programs, signs, or newsletters, the best-size type for these items is 18 point for residents who are visually impaired. For maximum readability, avoid highlighting text with bright-colored markers, which make reading more difficult for the visually impaired person because they diminish contrast. It is also good to avoid printing on colored paper or shiny materials, which also diminish readability.

For more information about making print more readable, see Appendix C, Tips for Print Readability.

TALKING BOOKS

The Talking Book Program is a national program to provide recorded books for individuals who are blind or visually impaired or who are physically disabled and cannot turn the pages of a book. It is provided by the National Library Service for the Blind and Physically Handicapped, part of the Library of Congress (see Appendix B). Books were originally recorded on records but are now recorded on tape. A tremendous variety of titles are available.

Talking books and a special tape machine on which to play them are available free of charge through a local or regional library for persons who are blind. (See the Resources section for phone number of the National Library Service.) Many vision rehabilitation agencies have application forms that require an authorizing signature to certify that the individual is sufficiently visually impaired or physically impaired to benefit from the program. Authorizing professionals include physicians, optometrists, ophthalmalogists, educators, social workers, librarians, rehabilitation teachers, or counselors. Many public libraries also have these forms.

Each month, users of the program can select from a catalog of available books and magazines or can request that titles in various categories such as mystery, science fiction, romance, or business be sent to them each month.

Facilities that have residents who are visually impaired can subscribe to the program by getting in touch with their state or regional Library for the Blind and Physically Handicapped.

OTHER BOOKS ON TAPE

Many current books are now available commercially on tape at most bookstores for the general public. These tapes do not require a special player, and they typically cost approximately what the print book costs.

Congratulations! You have reached the end of Lesson 9. Now go on to the Key Points to review what you have learned in this lesson.

KEY POINTS IN LESSON 9

Reading Techniques

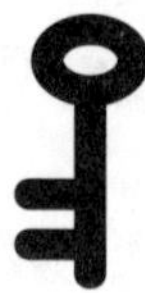

1. Task lighting and nonglare lighting are essential for reading.
2. Large-print materials (18 point or larger) may be helpful to the older resident. Encourage the use of large-print materials in your facility.
3. Residents with vision loss may be able to use reading devices such as magnifiers and CCTVs. These should be prescribed by a low vision specialist.
4. Residents may need encouragement to use their reading devices and may need to practice.
5. Residents who cannot read or who have difficulty reading with a device may prefer to use talking books, which are available for persons who qualify due to visual or physical disability.

LEARNING ACTIVITIES

Try the following activities to practice what you have learned in this lesson. Some of the activities involve the use of simulators—glasses that simulate different types of vision loss. (See Appendix B for sources of vision simulators.) It is important to work in pairs while doing these exercises. One person uses the simulators while the other watches for safety and provides feedback.

Familiarize yourself with different types of reading devices and how to use them (see catalogs in Appendix B).

You may wish to try out some of the devices using the vision simulators.

☑ SELF-CHECK

Indicate whether each statement is true (T) or false (F) in the space provided. Check Appendix A for the answers. Then go back and review any statements you may have missed.

______ 1. Task lighting is important for reading.

______ 2. Talking books are a good solution for residents who cannot read large print or hold a book and turn the pages.

______ 3. A CCTV is a useful low vision device for seeing pictures as well as printed material.

LESSON 10

Writing Techniques

GOAL

To teach a resident who is visually impaired to write using several kinds of writing guides and easier-to-see writing utensils.

OBJECTIVE

At the end of the lesson, you will know about writing guides and utensils, and you will be able to instruct the resident to write using writing guides and a felt-tip pen.

TEACH Principles

When teaching a resident about the different options for writing, use the five TEACH principles for working successfully with a resident who is visually impaired:

T—Talk to the resident about writing.

E—Encourage the resident to try writing.

A—Assess the resident's writing needs.

C—"Can do" is the motto for each resident.

H—Help the resident to become independent in writing.

Teaching Writing

An older person's writing skills may diminish at the same time as reading skills decrease if he or she is losing vision. This can make it difficult for a resident not only to write letters but also to take care of such everyday tasks as writing checks or making shopping lists. As with reading, there are several solutions to make writing easier for a resident. These include using

- contrast
- writing guides
- adapted writing tools
- task lighting (a light source such as a gooseneck lamp which shines directly on the writing area)

You can help the resident write more independently using these solutions.

Contrast

If there is not enough contrast between paper and writing surface, the paper edges may seem to disappear. Putting a solid-color place mat or a darker piece of paper under the writing paper can increase contrast and make the paper more visible. Contrast can also be achieved by putting the paper on a dark-colored clipboard.

White paper may cause glare; therefore, ivory-colored paper may be easier for residents to work with than white.

Writing Guides

Various writing guides or templates are available that can make it possible for the older person to independently sign his or her name, address an envelope, or write a check. These are guides for writing that use a cutout space or raised lines to help the writer stay on the line or in place. Writing guides are typically made of dark cardboard or similar materials so that they provide contrast. Common types of writing guides include signature, envelope, and check writing guides, in addition to handwriting guides.

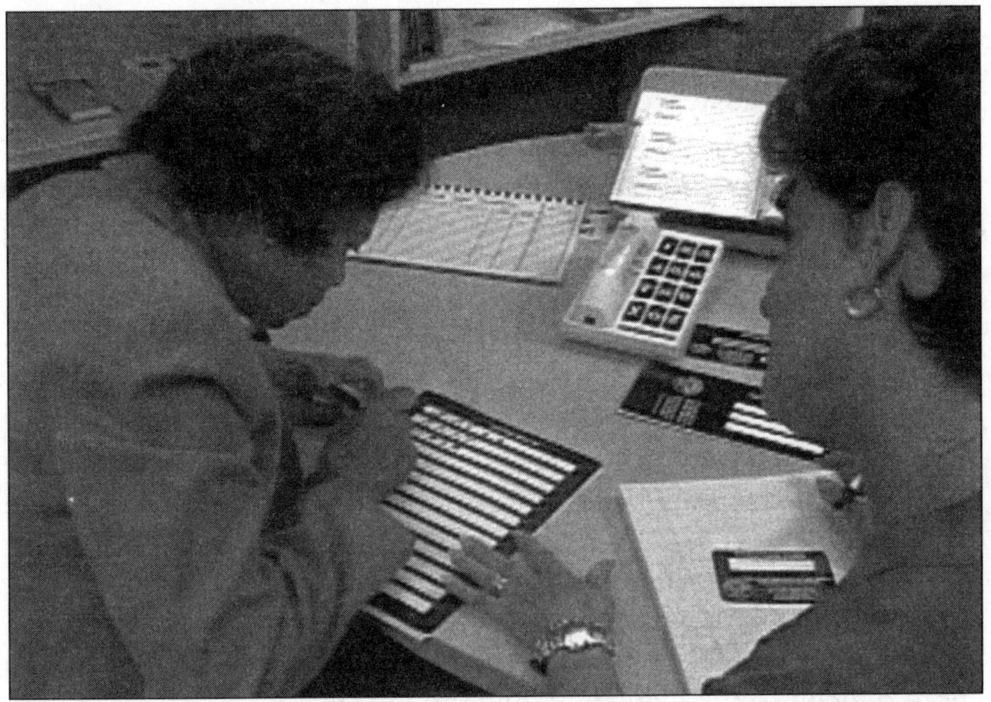
AMERICAN FOUNDATION FOR THE BLIND

Writing guides provide a space for writing that residents can feel. Different types can help residents write letters, write checks, and sign their name.

These guides can be made easily by using card stock or poster-board paper in a dark color to create contrast with the white or light-colored page on which they are placed. Depending on the purpose of the template, a window can be cut of the appropriate size and in the right place. The template can be turned on the angle at which the older person typically writes for comfort. The guides are also available for purchase through catalogs listed in Appendix B.

Adapted Writing Tools

Making sure the resident has the right tools to write with can make a lot of difference. Using regular lined paper can help an older person who still has some good usable vision to write straight and on the line. For residents with low vision, paper with extra-bold lines can make writing even easier. Bold-line paper is available from the catalogs listed in Appendix B.

A common problem is that the older person may manage to write, take notes, and write down telephone numbers but cannot read back what he or she has written. Writing with dark felt-tip pens, markers, or gel pens, primarily black, can make it easier for the older person to read back what he or she has written. Felt-tip pens and markers should be tested because some bleed through the paper. For example, the Sanford 20/20 Easy-to-Read Pen is a dark and thick felt-tip pen that is easier for residents to see. These can be purchased from the catalogs of low vision devices listed in Appendix B. Flair felt-tip pens and especially those with a bit more width are available in most office supply stores and can also be helpful when a 20/20 pen is not available.

Other Methods of Communicating

If an older resident has typing skills, it is sometimes easier for the older person to write a letter by typewriter or computer. Some residents may still have a typewriter. The disadvantage is that he or she may have difficulty reading the letter back to himself or herself. Using a larger-size type, which is easy to do on the computer, can help. Typing in all caps is never recommended. It makes it even more difficult to distinguish among the letters.

Increasing numbers of older people are learning computer skills. Residents can learn to use large-print screen magnifiers, computer programs which increase the size of text on the screen. Some will also be able to learn to work with a computer that is able to read the words on the screen aloud, known as *speech output* or *synthetic speech*.

Another way to communicate with others is to send a letter recorded on an audio cassette to other people who will record their messages in return. Cassettes can be mailed without charge using a program of the U.S. Postal Service known as Free Matter for the Blind and Other Physically Handicapped Persons.

Persons who receive talking books, who have been certified as legally blind, who are unable to read or unable to use standard printed material as a result of physical limitations, or who have a reading disability are eligible for Free Matter for the Blind service.

Individuals who meet eligibility requirements may receive the following types of reading matter:

- reading matter in braille or 14-point or larger type and musical scores (but no advertisements)
- sound reproductions
- paper, records, tapes, and other material for the production of reading matter, musical scores, or sound reproductions
- reproducers or parts of them for sound reproductions, braillewriters, typewriters, educational or other materials or

devices, or parts thereof, used for writing by, or adapted for use of, a blind person or a person who has a physical impairment

Eligible individuals may send without charge letters in braille or in 14-point or larger type or in the form of sound recordings, only if they contain no advertising and are unsealed. Letters that are handwritten, or printed or typed in a type size smaller than 14 points, may not be sent free. For additional details of this service, contact your post office.

Congratulations! You have reached the end of Lesson 10. Now go on to the key points to review what you have learned in this lesson.

KEY POINTS IN LESSON 10

Writing Techniques

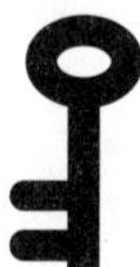

1. Use contrast between paper and writing surface.
2. Writing devices include:
   - ➤ writing guides or templates
   - ➤ bold-line paper
   - ➤ dark felt-tip pens
3. Task lighting may be helpful.

LEARNING ACTIVITIES

Try the following activities to practice what you have learned in this lesson. Some of the activities involve the use of simulators—glasses that simulate different types of vision loss. (See Appendix B for sources of vision simulators.) It is important to work in pairs while doing these exercises. One person uses the simulators while the other watches for safety and provides feedback.

Using the simulators, practice signing your name with a writing template and felt-tip pen.

Do the same using bold-line paper and a felt-tip pen.

☑ SELF-CHECK

Indicate whether each statement is true (T) or false (F) in the space provided. Check Appendix A for the answers. Then go back and review any statements you may have missed.

______ 1. Using black felt-tip pens such as the Sanford 20/20 brand can help a resident with a visual impairment write more legibly and to possibly see what he or she has written.

______ 2. A signature guide can be used to enable a resident to write his or her name in a letter or on a check.

LESSON 11

Using Large-Print and Talking Devices

GOAL

To show a resident who is visually impaired large-print and talking devices that can help the resident with balancing a checkbook, keeping up with addresses, and other personal tasks.

OBJECTIVE

By the end of this lesson, you will be able to familiarize a resident who is visually impaired with useful large-print and talking devices, such as talking calculators.

TEACH Principles

As you review large-print and talking devices with the residents, use the five TEACH principles for working successfully with a resident who is visually impaired:

T—Talk to the resident about large-print and talking devices.

E—Encourage the resident to try out the devices.

A—Assess the resident's need for some of the devices.

C—"Can do" is the motto for each resident.

H—Help the resident to learn to use the devices of his or her choice.

Large-Print and Talking Devices

A great many specialized devices are available to help people who are blind or visually impaired with financial management (such as writing checks and keeping their checkbook) as well as everyday tasks such as looking up telephone numbers and checking their weight. These may be ordinary household devices and tools, such as calculators, clocks, or scales with large numbers or labels for ease of use, or they may be designed to "speak" a measurement or reading to the user. These devices are available from the catalogs listed in Appendix B.

Financial Management

Being able to manage their own money and keep track of their finances is very important to older people and helps them continue to feel independent. You can show residents who are visually impaired devices such as large-print or talking calculators that can help them balance their checkbooks and keep track of their spending.

CALCULATORS

Depending on the resident's degree of vision, the resident can be taught to use either a large-print or talking calculator. Such devices are available commercially and through the catalogs listed in Appendix B.

SELECTING AN APPROPRIATE CALCULATOR

You will need to go over the features of each type of calculator with the resident to determine which will best suit the resident's needs. Some talking calculators feature female voices and others male voices. Some have volume control, earphones, and/or large liquid crystal displays (LCDs). Some operate on battery power and/or solar power; others have a battery and an AC adapter. Some have printouts. There are also desktop and portable models.

FAMILIARIZING THE RESIDENT WITH KEYS AND FUNCTIONS

Regardless of the type of calculator used, you will need to work with the resident to familiarize him or her with the keys. Most of the keyboard numbering systems organize numbers using 3 columns.

Residents need to learn to use the "home row" technique. This means placing the fingers in the same place on the calculator keypad before they use it so that they are oriented to the location of all the keys. They should place their first three fingers on the three keys of the middle row across: 4, 5, 6. Most calculators have a tactile marking on the number 5 key, which lets the user know where his or her fingers are on the numbered keypad. You should mark the 5 key for the resident if the calculator has no tactile marking.

BALANCING A CHECKBOOK

If the resident is using the calculator to balance a checkbook, he or she may need a large-print check and deposit register to maintain records and balance the checkbook. These are available from most banks upon request or can be ordered through the catalogs listed in Appendix B.

It is sometimes useful to use a template such as a writing guide to move down the page of the register to help the resident stay on the right line. As discussed in Lesson 10, there are several varieties of templates available. Some residents may also wish to use a bold-line pen or marker to make their entries. This makes reading entries easier.

TRACKING SPENDING

For residents with low vision who want to keep track of their spending or other items, writing the expenditures on easy-to-read bold-line paper may be helpful. Bold-line paper comes in single sheets or in notebook style. Some residents may wish to use a tape recorder to track their expenditures.

Other Useful Large-Print Devices

There are a number of other large-print devices that are available to help the resident with everyday tasks. These are available through the catalogs listed in Appendix B. They include

- large-print calendars
- easy-to-read weight scales with large, lit numbers

- large-print address books
- large-print rulers and tape measures
- easy-to-read blood pressure monitors

Other Useful Talking Devices

A number of talking devices are also available. These can be ordered through the catalogs listed in Appendix B. They include

- talking weight scales for weighing a person
- talking caller ID for the telephones
- talking blood pressure monitors
- talking glucose monitors
- talking digital thermometers

Congratulations! You have reached the end of Lesson 11. Now go on to the Key Points to review what you have learned in this lesson.

KEY POINTS IN LESSON 11

Using Large-Print and Talking Devices

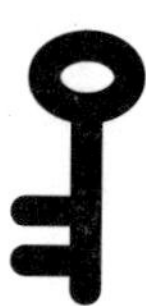

1. A number of devices are available to help the resident with a visual impairment. Some include
    - large-print and talking calculators
    - large-print checkbooks
    - large-print calendars
    - large-print address books
    - large-print rulers
    - talking weight scales
2. A number of other devices are available to meet many of the needs of residents. Review the catalogs listed in Appendix B to familiarize yourself with other products.

LEARNING ACTIVITIES

Try the following activities to practice what you have learned in this lesson. Some of the activities involve the use of simulators—glasses that simulate different types of vision loss. (See Appendix B for sources of vision simulators.) It is important to work in pairs while doing these exercises. One person uses the simulators while the other watches for safety and provides feedback.

- Try using both large-print and talking calculators using the simulators.
- Try explaining how to use the keyboard of a talking calculator to another staff member who is using simulators.
- Practice using other devices.

SELF-CHECK

Indicate whether each statement is true (T) or false (F) in the space provided. Check Appendix A for the answers. Then go back and review any statements you may have missed.

______ 1. Talking calculators are available now in many different styles and with many different features.

______ 2. Very few other devices are available to help individuals with visual impairments.

LESSON 12 Using a Telephone

GOAL

To instruct the resident in how to use a telephone effectively.

OBJECTIVE

You will be able to demonstrate how to teach a resident to dial a phone and to solicit assistance from an operator.

TEACH Principles

As you work with the resident on using the telephone, use the five TEACH principles for working successfully with a resident who is visually impaired:

T—**Talk** to the resident about the use of the telephone.

E—**Encourage** the resident to use the telephone.

A—**Assess** the resident's ability to use the telephone.

C—"**Can do**" is the motto for each resident.

H—Help the resident to learn to use the telephone at least for emergency calls.

Using a Telephone

Most telephones now are push button. In the rare instance of a rotary phone, a large-print overlay can be placed on the dial to help the resident with low vision see the dial. Push-button telephones with large numerals are available commercially, through telephone companies, or through catalogs listed in Appendix B.

In learning to dial by touch, it is critical for the resident to learn the positions of the numbers. The left column has numbers 1,4,7; the middle has 2,5,8,0; and the right column has 3,6,9. The home row keys of 4,5,6 should be memorized and used to find the other keys.

The resident may find it helpful to use three fingers—index, middle, and ring—while navigating up and down the numbered keypad. On most newer, American-made phones, the resident can look for a tactile marking on the number 5. If the 5 is not marked, it may be helpful to the resident to mark it with Hi-Marks (see Lesson 1).

To enable residents to call 911 or 0 for operator assistance, you may want to ask the resident to practice calling these numbers.

Programmable phones can now be obtained. A resident can program or have someone else program the telephone numbers he or she calls most often. The resident can then reach these numbers by pressing only one function button or a two-digit number assigned to the telephone number. Voice-recognition telephones are also now available but are not always reliable.

Operator Assistance

Operator assistance is available free of charge for people who are visually impaired by completing an application with your telephone service provider. The local telephone company will provide information and applications. This service can be useful to residents who feel uncomfortable using the phone or have trouble finding the right numbers.

Maintaining a List of Telephone Numbers

Helping residents keep their address books or list of telephone numbers up-to-date and legible is important to enable them to stay in communication with their friends and relatives.

In the writing lesson, Lesson 10, you learned about bold-line paper and writing templates. If able to see lined paper and read bold numbers, the resident may want to write his or her own list of telephone numbers using a felt-tip pen.

An alternative technique for keeping a telephone list is to help the resident develop a cassette recording of the telephone list, including important names and numbers.

Congratulations! You have reached the end of Lesson 12. Now go on to the Key Points to review what you have learned in this lesson.

KEY POINTS IN LESSON 12

Using a Telephone

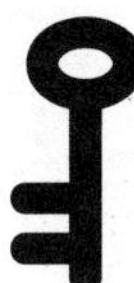

1. Most residents can learn to use a push-button telephone by memorizing the keypad and practicing dialing.
2. Phones and phone dial pads are available in large print.
3. Operator assistance is available free of charge for residents with visual impairments through application.
4. Phone lists in large print or on tape may be helpful to the resident.

LEARNING ACTIVITIES

Try the following activities to practice what you have learned in this lesson. Some of the activities involve the use of simulators—glasses that simulate different types of vision loss. (See Appendix B for sources of vision simulators.) It is important to work in pairs while doing these exercises. One person uses the simulators while the other watches for safety and provides feedback.

- Practice dialing a phone using the simulators.
- Practice teaching someone to dial a phone using simulators.

☑ SELF-CHECK

Indicate whether each statement is true (T) or false (F) in the space provided. Check Appendix A for the answers. Then go back and review any statements you may have missed.

______ 1. The resident with a visual impairment can apply to receive free directory assistance.

______ 2. Large-print push-button phones are available for individuals who can read large print.

LESSON 13 Telling Time

GOAL

To teach the older resident to tell time.

OBJECTIVE

At the end of this lesson, you will be able to identify several ways to tell time and to teach the most appropriate method to the resident.

TEACH Principles

As you work with the resident to tell time, use the five TEACH principles for working successfully with a resident who is visually impaired:

T—**Talk** to the resident about telling time.

E—**Encourage** the resident to try telling time.

A—**Assess** the resident's ability to use a variety of time-telling devices.

C—"**Can do**" is the motto for each resident.

H—Help the resident to learn to use the devices of his or her choice.

Using Large-Print Watches and Clocks

Many older residents with visual impairments will be able to see large-print watches and clocks that have black numbers on a white background. Remember, the hands tell the time. The contrast and size of the hands are more important than the size of the numbers.

Dark hands on a white surface work well for many older people who are visually impaired. However, white hands and numbers on a black background work best for some people. Both types of large-print watches and clocks are available commercially through the catalogs listed in Appendix B.

Many types of watchbands are available now. For older residents, especially those who are visually impaired, expansion bands may be easier to use than those that buckle.

Using Talking Watches and Clocks

For residents who cannot see a watch or clock face, a talking watch or clock is a good alternative as long as the older person's hearing is still good. Test the talking watch for sound quality. A resident with a hearing impairment may have difficulty with the sound of some talking watches. Both male and female voices are available, as well as different languages.

Keep in mind that talking watches can be difficult to set without sighted assistance. Some may have small and hard-to-use buttons, and the batteries are hard for the resident to replace alone. You may need to provide assistance in completing these tasks. Talking watches and clocks are also available now through the catalogs listed in Appendix B.

Using a Braille Watch or Clock

Some residents who have trouble reading even a large-print watch may prefer to use a braille watch or clock. They do not need to know how to read braille to use these watches. Braille watches and clocks have an open face with raised dots placed where the numbers would usually be, for example:

12:00—three vertical dots ⋮

3:00 and 9:00—two horizontal dots • •

6:00—two vertical dots :

Other hours—one dot •

To tell time with a braille watch, the resident should feel the direction of the large and small hands in relation to the dots. Have the resident start by feeling the hands at the center of the watch and then tracing each hand outward to the numbers. The resident may find the index finger to be the most sensitive and therefore may want to use it for this task.

For example, if the large and small hands are both pointed at three vertical dots, the resident will know it is 12 o'clock. If the large hand is pointed at three vertical dots and the small hand at two vertical dots, the resident will know it is 6 o'clock.

Congratulations! You have reached the end of Lesson 13. Now go on to the Key Points to review what you have learned in this lesson.

KEY POINTS IN LESSON 13

Telling Time

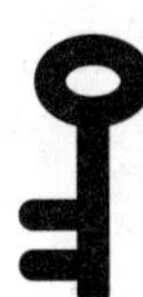

1. Most residents can learn to use a talking watch or clock.
2. Watches and clocks are available with large-print faces.
3. Residents may need help setting a talking watch or clock and with changing the batteries.

LEARNING ACTIVITIES

Try the following activities to practice what you have learned in this lesson. Some of the activities involve the use of simulators—glasses that simulate different types of vision loss. (See Appendix B for sources of vision simulators.) It is important to work in pairs while doing these exercises. One person uses the simulators while the other watches and provides feedback.

Special Skill Areas

O‑π Practice reading a large-print watch while wearing simulators.

O‑π Practice setting and listening to a talking clock while wearing simulators.

☑ SELF-CHECK

Indicate whether each statement is true (T) or false (F) in the space provided. Check Appendix A for the answers. Then go back and review any statements you may have missed.

______ 1. Residents with visual impairments can tell time using a talking watch or clock.

______ 2. Braille watches can only be used by persons who read braille.

LESSON 14

Identifying Money

GOAL

To show a resident who is visually impaired how to identify coins, maintain a folding system for paper money, and identify differently folded bills.

OBJECTIVES

- ➤ By the end of this lesson, you will be familiar with a system for identifying bills and differentiating among coins tactilely.
- ➤ You will be able to assist a resident with steps to identify money.

TEACH Principles

As you work with the resident to identify money, use the five TEACH principles for working successfully with a resident who is visually impaired:

T—**Talk** to the resident about identifying money.

E—**Encourage** the resident to try to identify coins.

A—**Assess** the resident's ability to identify coins and fold bills.

C—"**Can do**" is the motto for each resident.

H—**Help** the resident to learn to identify money if he or she wishes to learn.

Learning to Identify Money

Being able to handle money and make one's own purchases is an important part of feeling like an independent adult. It can be difficult for a person who is visually impaired to tell different denominations of money apart, especially bills, but there are systems they can use to make this much easier.

Differentiating Coins

Coins can be differentiated by their size, their edges, and their thickness. Residents with low vision will probably be able to see the difference in color between the copper penny and the other silver coins.

CLUES FOR DIFFERENTIATING COINS

SIZE Since the dime is the smallest, this leaves the penny, nickel, and quarter to distinguish. These are the hardest to differentiate.

THICKNESS The nickel is the thickest among the coins.

EDGES The penny and the nickel have smooth edges and the dime and the quarter have rough edges.

When teaching the resident to identify coins, use the following steps:

STEPS TO IDENTIFYING COINS

STEP 1 Lay out coins. To assist the resident in identifying money, place a penny, nickel, dime, and quarter in the resident's hand one at a time. The dollar coin can also be used when available.

STEP 2 Feel the coins. Have the resident finger the coins. Ask the resident to observe the size, edges, and thickness of the coins.

STEP 3 Try to identify coins. Ask the resident to identify the coins that he or she is able to distinguish.

STEP 4 Practice. Work with the resident to identify the coins that he or she was unable to identify by using the size, edges, and thickness cues described.

Folding Money for Identification

A folding system can be utilized to help a resident identify paper money, which has no physically distinguishing features. In the folding method, each denomination of bill is folded in a different way, which can be easily felt by the resident.

First ask if the resident is currently using any method to identify bills. If so, have the resident show you the system. If the system is working for the resident, he or she can continue to use it. You may be able to help with additional suggestions for the resident's system.

If the resident does not have a system or needs some suggestions, you can describe the folding method as a means of identifying paper money. The following is a typical method of folding bills.

TYPICAL METHOD OF FOLDING BILLS

Someone must identify the denominations to the person who is visually impaired.

- Leave $1 bills unfolded.
- Fold $5 bills by width. (Folding in this manner will make the $1 bills and $5 bills taller in the billfold.)
- Fold $10 bills lengthwise.

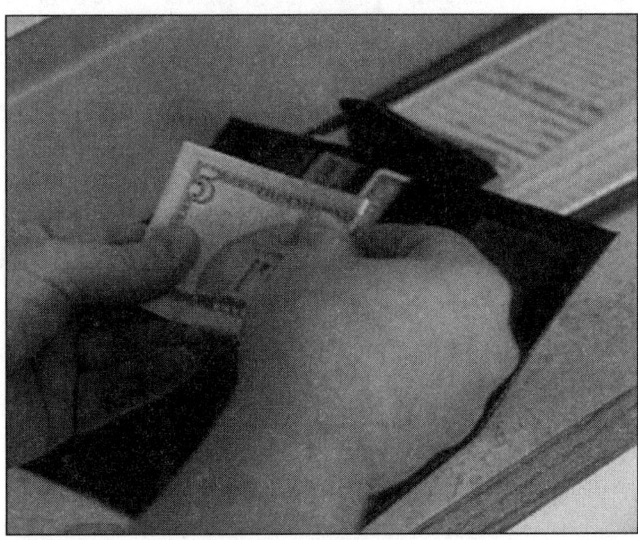

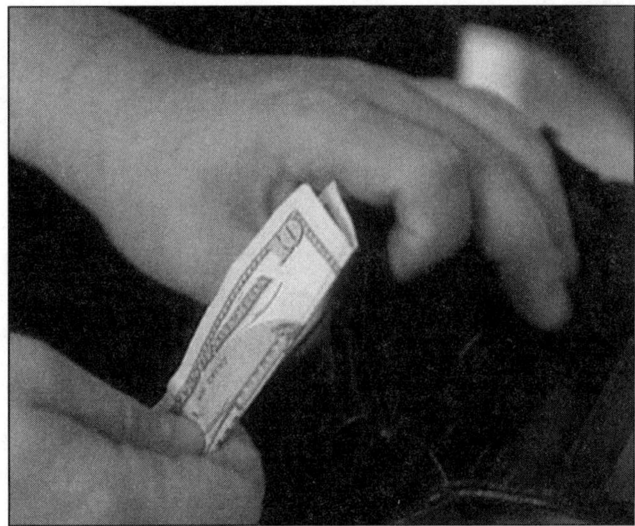

AMERICAN FOUNDATION FOR THE BLIND

One way of keeping track of money is to fold bills of different denominations in different ways.

- Fold $20 bills both lengthwise and by width, or just leave them open, and place them in the bottom or back of a wallet, since they may be the least frequently used denomination.

A wallet with four separate bill compartments is available from some of the catalogs in Appendix B. This wallet enables the resident to keep bills separated easily.

PRACTICING IDENTIFYING MONEY

To help the resident practice the folding method of identifying bills, try some of the following exercises.

- Fold some bills and put them in an envelope with several coins. Ask the resident to open the envelope and tell you what is inside.
- Have the resident fold some bills and put them in a wallet. Role-play being in a grocery store and have the resident pretend to pay for something.
- Give both bills and coins as change and ask the resident to identify them.

HANDLING MONEY SAFELY

In addition to learning how to identify their money, residents who are visually impaired can make use of certain practices to keep their money as safe as possible. Suggest that the resident announce the denomination of the currency used in a transaction and request that the clerk announce the denominations of the bills given back in change. As each bill is identified aloud, the resident can then fold each bill. Bills should be put away in a billfold as soon as possible to avoid confusion and the possibility of losing them.

Also suggest that the resident use the denomination of currency closest to the amount of the transaction. This will minimize the chance of being shortchanged.

Congratulations! You have reached the end of Lesson 14. Now go on to the Key Points to review what you have learned in this lesson.

KEY POINTS IN LESSON 14
Identifying Money

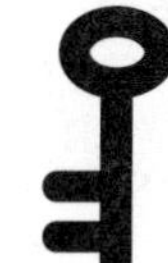

1. Coins can be differentiated by size, edges, and thickness.
2. Bills should be folded in different ways to help in identification.

LEARNING ACTIVITIES

Try the following activities to practice what you have learned in this lesson. Some of the activities involve the use of simulators—glasses that simulate different types of vision loss. (See Appendix B for sources of vision simulators.) It is important to work in pairs while doing these exercises. One person uses the simulators while the other watches for safety and provides feedback.

- Close your eyes and practice identifying coins.
- With your eyes closed, try to make change for a dollar.
- Close your eyes and practice folding bills. Have someone mix up the bills for you and attempt to identify them.

SELF-CHECK

Indicate whether each statement is true (T) or false (F) in the space provided. Check Appendix A for the answers. Then go back and review any statements you may have missed.

______ 1. Coins always have smooth edges.

______ 2. Folding bills in different ways is a good technique to use to identify them.

LESSON 15 Caring for Clothing

GOAL

To teach the resident to keep clothing organized so that it is easy to identify and launder.

OBJECTIVE

At the end of the lesson, you will be able to show the resident techniques to sort and organize clothes.

Teach Principles

As you review methods of identifying and organizing clothing with the residents, use the five TEACH principles for working successfully with a resident who is visually impaired:

T—**Talk** to the resident about organizing and caring for clothing.

E—**Encourage** the resident to develop a system of identifying clothes.

A—Assess the resident's ability to identify clothes.

C—"Can do" is the motto for each resident.

H—Help the resident to learn to develop a system for identifying clothes if he or she wishes to do so.

Managing Clothing Care

There are several factors to consider when residents are trying to independently manage clothing care. The first is that the resident should be able to identify each clothing item, particularly the color, so they can be properly matched. You can also show residents techniques to help them with laundering their clothes.

Identifying Clothing

Residents may have trouble finding particular articles of clothing that they want to wear or distinguishing the color of clothing in order to match outfits. You can teach them techniques to help with identifying clothing. Some articles of clothing have distinctive elements that can be identified by touch, such as textured fabric or buttons. For other items that do not have a ready-made way to identify them, sorting, labeling, and organizing are important elements to clothing management.

SORTING

Clothes that are frequently worn together can be hung together as an outfit, such as a skirt and blouse, a turtleneck and pants, or a dress and jacket. This makes it easier to locate these items.

Identifying and matching socks can be particularly difficult. Sock clips can be used to keep matching socks together. The resident can clip a pair of socks together upon taking them off. They can go through the washer and dryer this way and remain matched. Sock clips are available commercially as well as in the specialty catalogs listed in Appendix B. Safety pins can also be used for this purpose.

Another trick is to own only all-white socks and all-black socks, for example, which are easy to distinguish from each other but can be matched with any other sock of that color.

LABELING

Another way to identify clothing is to label it. For example, a resident may have two or more of the same article of clothing in different colors, such as the same brand of slacks in black, navy, and brown. These may be hard to distinguish, since they are all dark colors. There are a number of ways to label clothing.

You can help the resident set up a personalized color identification system. For example, you can put a safety pin on the inside label of the navy pants pointing horizontally, a safety pin pointing vertically on the brown pair, and nothing on the black pair. Have the resident assist you in developing the labeling system so that it will be easy for the resident to remember and use it.

You can also use safety pins to develop a system for matching clothing. For example, all clothes with one pin can be worn with all other clothes with one pin, clothes with two pins can be worn with other clothes with two pins, and so on.

Small metal braille labels can be purchased to label clothing (see Appendix B for catalogs). Each label is just one or two letters that the resident can learn to recognize tactilely (by touch) without having to learn to read braille. However, some tactile methods of identification are difficult for the resident who has diabetic retinopathy because of the neuropathy associated with diabetes (loss of sensitivity in the fingertips). In these cases, other larger or more easily identifiable labeling is needed.

For example, one commercial system (available from the catalogs in Appendix B) uses plastic tags in different shapes. You can also identify clothing with handwritten labels in large print written with a bold marker. The labels can be left on the hanger when the garment is worn.

ROBERT HAKALSKI/VISUAL MACHINERY

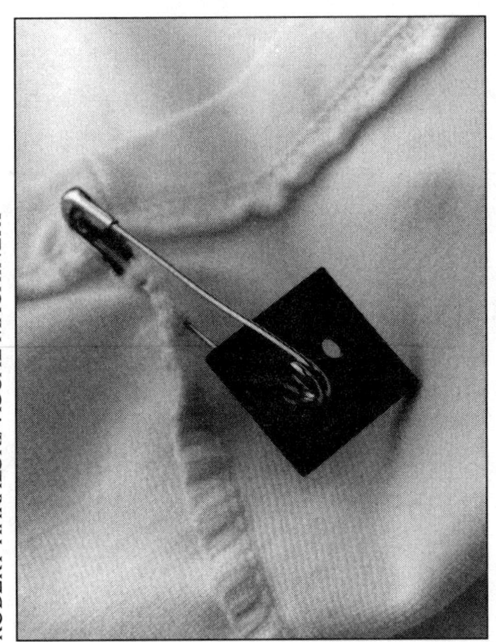

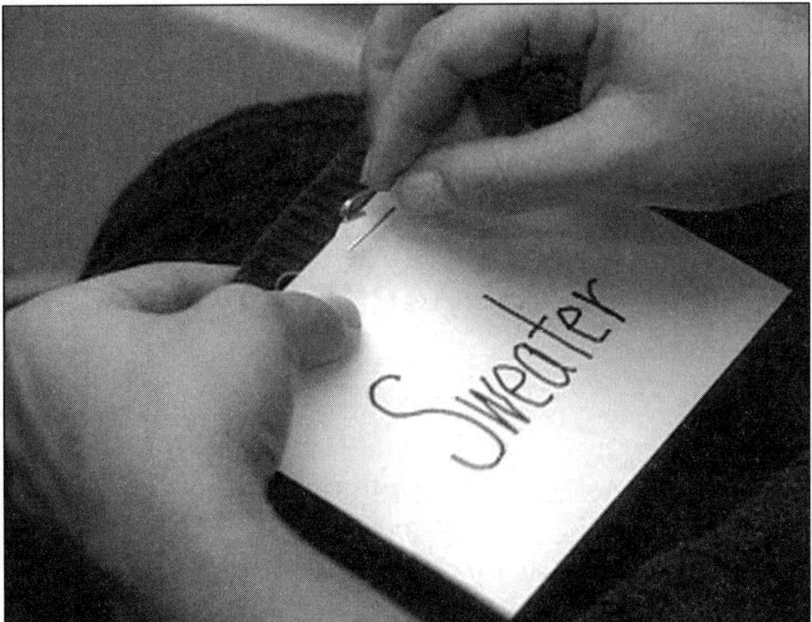

AMERICAN FOUNDATION FOR THE BLIND

Two ways to label clothing: a commercial system using different shaped plastic tags, and a hand-written tag in large, dark print.

ORGANIZING DRAWERS AND CLOSETS

For residents to be able to find the clothing they want to wear, it is important to organize drawers and closets so there is a place for everything and to always put clothes back in the same place.

Dividers can be used in drawers to separate items and keep them in order. For example, the white socks could be placed on one side of the divider and the black socks on the other.

Plastic bags or plastic shoe boxes can be used as inexpensive organizers. Egg cartons and fishing tackle boxes are great containers for earrings and other jewelry.

Doing Laundry

If residents do their own laundry, there are several elements involved. These include setting the dials on the washer and dryer, measuring and pouring laundry detergent, and sorting laundry whites and darks.

SORTING LAUNDRY

The easiest way to sort laundry is to immediately place white and dark clothing each in separate laundry bags when they are taken off and are ready for laundering. This eliminates sorting at washing time.

MEASURING LAUNDRY DETERGENT

Use a measuring cup to measure dry and liquid laundry detergents. Measure over the washer so that any excess will still go in the wash. The resident might also try detergent tablets. These are premeasured tablets with detergent, and depending on the brand, they may have other laundry ingredients such as fabric softener or stain fighters.

MARKING AND SETTING CONTROLS

Washer and dryer settings can be marked with a substance called Hi-Marks, which forms a raised marking when it dries (see Lesson 1). The resident can then feel when the dial points to the correct setting.

Rather than marking each setting, only the most frequently used settings need to be marked for easier identification. Then the resident will only need to memorize the essential settings.

Congratulations! You have reached the end of Lesson 15. Now go on to the Key Points to review what you have learned in this lesson.

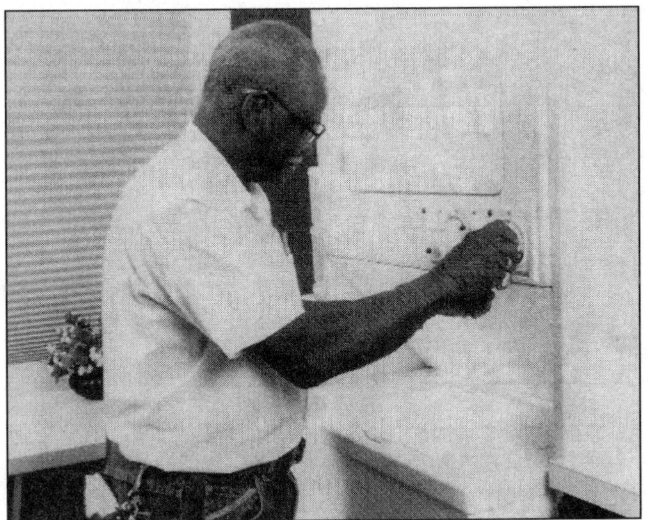

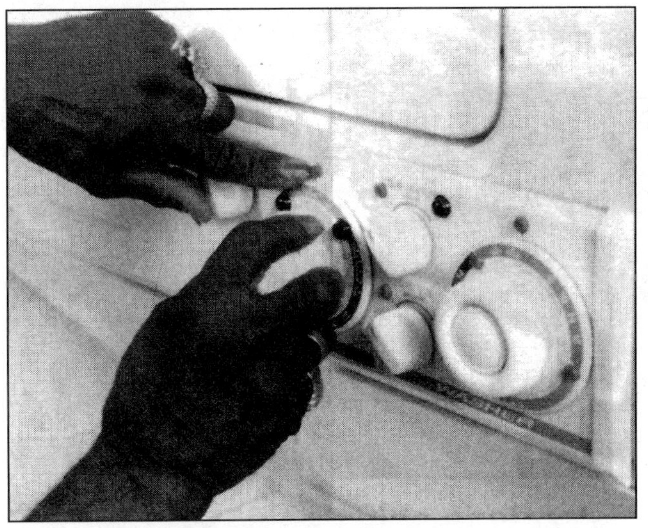

ROBERT HAKALSKI/VISUAL MACHINERY

The most commonly used settings on a washing machine or dryer can be marked with a raised substance such as Hi-Marks so residents can feel when the dials point to the right setting.

KEY POINTS IN LESSON 15

Caring for Clothing

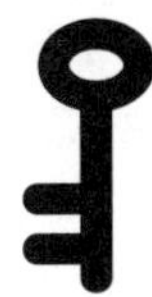

1. Create a system for identifying clothing. Key concepts include
   - sorting
   - organizing
   - labeling
2. For laundering clothes, key concepts include
   - sorting clothes as they are removed
   - using a measuring cup to measure laundry detergent
   - marking washer and dryer settings with a tactile marker

LEARNING ACTIVITIES

Try the following activities to practice what you have learned in this lesson. Some of the activities involve the use of simulators—glasses that simulate different types of vision loss. (See Appendix B for sources of vision simulators.) It is important to work in pairs while doing these exercises. One person uses the simulators while the other watches for safety and provides feedback.

Special Skill Areas

- Develop a system for sorting and labeling a few outfits.
- Ask another staff member to place these in a closet.
- Using simulators, try to put together an outfit to wear to work.

☑ SELF-CHECK

Indicate whether each statement is true (T) or false (F) in the space provided. Check Appendix A for the answers. Then go back and review any statements you may have missed.

______ 1. Clothes can be organized in a closet by using methods such as safety pins and/or clothing tags to differentiate colors.

______ 2. Using sock clips is one method to keep track of matching socks.

LESSON 16 Organizing Personal Items

GOAL

To teach the resident who is visually impaired ways in which to organize personal items.

OBJECTIVE

By the end of the lesson, you will be able to help a resident establish a system for organizing personal items.

TEACH Principles

As you review methods of organizing personal items with the residents, use the five TEACH principles for working successfully with a resident who is visually impaired:

T—Talk to the resident about organizing personal items.

E—Encourage the resident to try organizing personal items.

A—Assess the resident's ability to organize and locate items.

C—"Can do" is the motto for each resident.

H—Help the resident to learn to organize personal items if he or she wishes to do so.

Developing an Organizational System for Personal Items

Everyone has items that they frequently lose track of, such as eyeglasses, the remote control for the television, and personal items such as a hairbrush. This becomes even more of a concern when the individual can't use vision to search for these items. It is particularly important for residents who have visual impairments to keep their personal possessions organized so that they are easy to find.

You can help the resident set up a system that makes sense to the resident and will help keep things organized and easy to locate again. Keep items near where they are used. Establish a specific place for each item; for example, eyeglasses on the nightstand, a hair brush on the right-hand side of the dresser. The resident should try to return items to the same place each time. Items can be marked or labeled to help you and the resident remember the location and to encourage the resident to use the system.

TIPS FOR ORGANIZING PERSONAL ITEMS

- Create organization.
- Establish a place for each item.
- Always keep items in the same place every time.
- Return all items to their designated place as soon as you are finished using them.

Concerns about Rearranging Personal Items

All staff should know that when a resident is visually impaired, they should never move or rearrange the resident's personal items, as this will make it difficult for the resident to find them. In addition, neither the furniture in a resident's personal quarters nor the furniture in communal environments should be rearranged without informing the resident, as this can be disorienting and can make it hard for the resident to find his or her way around.

Congratulations! You have reached the end of Lesson 16. Now go on to the Key Points to review what you have learned in this lesson.

KEY POINTS IN LESSON 16

Organizing Personal Items

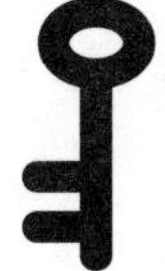

1. Help the resident create a system for keeping track of personal items. Key concepts include:
   - ➤ Create an organizational scheme.
   - ➤ Keep all items in the designated place.
   - ➤ Return all items to the designated place.
2. Do not rearrange items or furniture in a resident's environment without informing the resident.

LEARNING ACTIVITIES

Try the following activities to practice what you have learned in this lesson. Some of the activities involve the use of simulators—glasses that simulate different types of vision loss. (See Appendix B for sources of vision simulators.) It is important to work in pairs while doing these exercises. One person uses the simulators while the other watches for safety and provides feedback.

Think about where you keep your personal items, such as keys, watch, eyeglasses, remote controls, and hairbrush.

Think about logical places to keep these items so that they will not become lost.

Try this system and practice finding these items without looking.

SELF-CHECK

Indicate whether each statement is true (T) or false (F) in the space provided. Check Appendix A for the answers. Then go back and review any statements you may have missed.

______ 1. Keeping personal items in a designated place is a good idea for residents with visual impairments.

______ 2. You should not rearrange a resident's furniture or personal items without telling the resident.

LESSON 17 Safe Techniques in the Kitchen

GOAL

To teach the resident simple food preparation skills and techniques to operate safely and efficiently in the kitchen.

OBJECTIVE

By the end of the lesson, you will be able to show the resident how to carry out basic food preparation tasks safely, effectively, and efficiently.

TEACH Principles

As you review methods of basic food preparation with the resident, use the five TEACH principles for working successfully with a resident who is visually impaired:

T—Talk to the resident about safe food preparation.

E—Encourage the resident to try some safe food preparation techniques.

A—Assess the resident's kitchen area.

C—"Can do" is the motto for each resident.

H—Help the resident to learn about organizing and adapting the kitchen and preparing foods of his or her choice.

Working in the Kitchen

This lesson applies to those facilities where residents have their own kitchen. Some residents in these facilities are still interested in preparing simple meals or perhaps just a cup of tea or coffee. You can help them find out about certain techniques or specific aids and appliances available for older persons with visual impairments.

> **CAUTION:** Rehabilitation teachers are professionals who are specially trained to teach persons who are blind or visually impaired to cook safely. Residents who are interested in learning adapted cooking skills should be referred to a vision rehabilitation agency for further assistance by a rehabilitation teacher (see Appendix G).

There are a number of areas that need to be considered even before starting to work in the kitchen. These include lighting, safety, ways of organizing and labeling food so that it can be easily found, marking appliances for easy use, and using contrast for visibility in the kitchen. You can teach residents who are visually impaired simple techniques for cooking tasks such as measuring and pouring. Special devices are also available to help with many cooking tasks.

Lighting

Before starting to work with a resident on kitchen skills, you need to make sure the lighting in the kitchen is adequate and appropriate. Review Lesson 4 and use Appendix E, Creating a Functional Environment, and Appendix F, An Environmental Checklist, to review the lighting needs for a kitchen. Work with the resident and the management of the facility to make necessary changes. For example, task lighting placed in strategic areas may help the resident to better see the cooking task.

Safety

Discuss safety with the resident before beginning any sort of food preparation. There are a few basic principles that will make working in the kitchen much safer for residents who are visually impaired.

KITCHEN SAFETY PRINCIPLES

- Long oven mitts should always be worn when using the oven or other food heating appliances. These mitts minimize the chances of a resident burning an arm. They are available commercially as well as through the catalogs listed in Appendix B.
- Help the resident remember to keep all cabinet doors closed when not putting things in or taking them out. This will help the resident avoid hitting the head or shins.
- Teach the resident to turn the handles of cooking pots in toward the center line of the stove. This lessens the risk of knocking a pot off the stove and being injured.
- Make sure the resident knows to turn off oven and stove dials before removing food.

Organizing Items in a Kitchen

As described in Lesson 16, making sure every item is always put away in the same designated place helps people who are visually impaired to keep track of their belongings. This principle applies to the kitchen, too.

You can help the resident get organized by

- helping to clear away clutter and dispose of seldom-used and expired items
- organizing utensils in drawers with a method that makes sense to the resident and that the resident will use consistently. Make sure knives are put in a separate location from other utensils, so he or she doesn't encounter a sharp point or edge accidentally.
- hanging the most frequently used pots and pans on a pegboard within easy reach

Also work with the resident to develop a system that is meaningful to the resident to organize foods on cupboard shelves or in the refrigerator so that every type of food has its designated place. You can use large-print labels on the shelves, if the resident can read them, to indicate what belongs there. This will help family and friends to use the organization system. You can also set up different-colored labels or an alphabetical system for where to place cans on the shelves.

In addition, you can label the food items themselves, as suggested in the next section.

Organizing and Labeling Food

As soon as groceries are purchased, residents should label cans or frozen food so that they can identify them later. Any method that will help the resident remember what the can or product holds can be useful. The most important thing is to help develop a system that works for the resident.

Some common methods of labeling food are explained below.

- ➤ Magnetic letters, such as those sold for children, can be used to identify canned items.
- ➤ Large-print letters can be written on an unruled index card if the resident can see the print unaided or with a magnifier. Different-colored cards can be used to distinguish among categories of items.

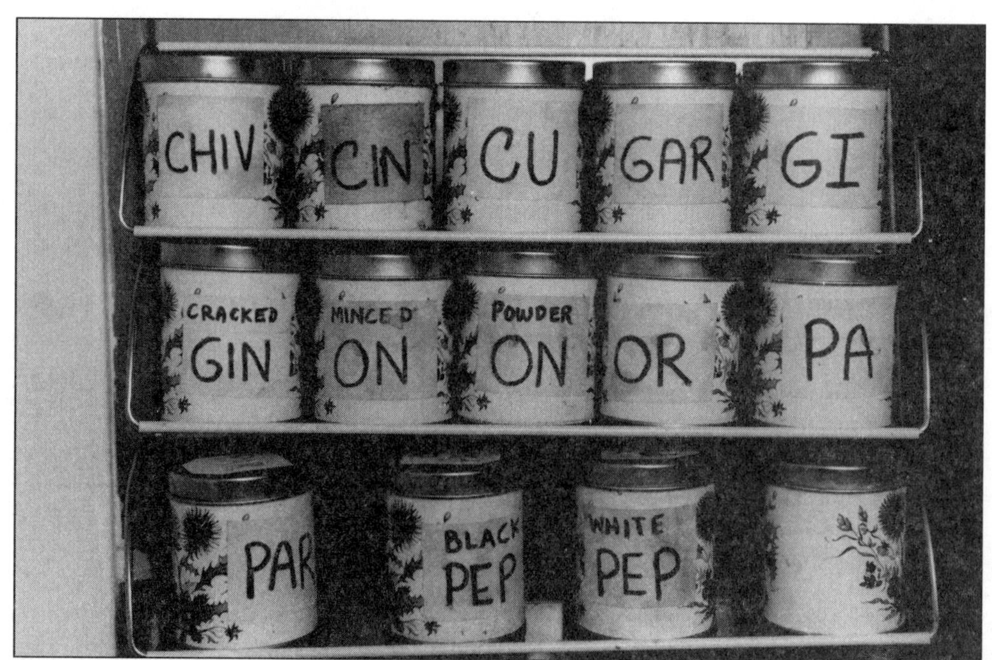

Large-print labels attached with rubber bands help to keep track of similar-looking items on the shelf.

- Colored twist ties can be used on plastic bags placed in a freezer to aid in organization.
- Different-colored plastic wrap or wraps with different textures, such as plastic and foil, can help with identification.
- Zip-lock plastic bags can be used with large print labels to organize frozen foods.

It is critical to insist that anyone who helps the resident put away groceries use the systems the resident has developed. The resident may feel intimidated by a well-meaning daughter or friend who "reorganizes" for the resident, but this change in the system may result in confusion and frustration for the resident.

Marking Appliances

It is often very difficult for a resident with a visual impairment to see the dials on a stove or other appliance. You can help the resident by marking the appliances that he or she uses with tactile marking substances (see Lesson 1).

Mark the oven or burner dial at the point the resident uses the most. For example, 350°F is a common setting for baking. Mark the stove and turn the knob until the mark on the dial matches the one on the stove. Hi-Marks, a product that is available commercially or through the catalogs listed in Appendix B, is one of the best products

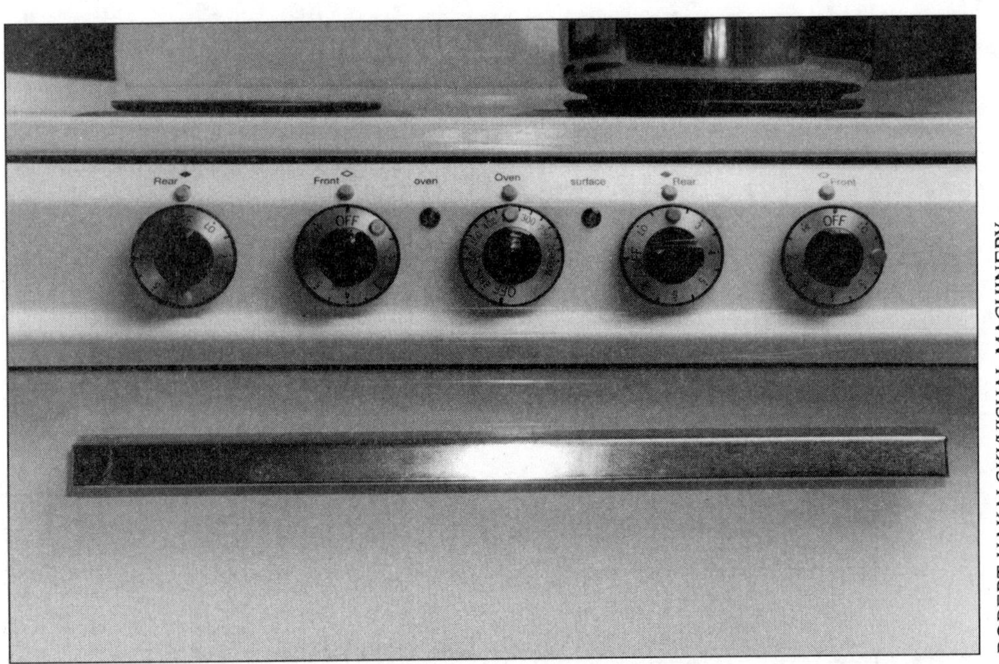

ROBERT HAKALSKI/VISUAL MACHINERY

Marking the stove with raised dots that have adhesive backs lets residents feel the most commonly used settings.

on the market for marking all sorts of appliances. It is durable and will usually stay on a stove or other appliance. Raised dots with adhesive backs are also sold. Other suggestions are glue and nail polish.

Mark any other appliance the resident plans to use, such as the stove, dishwasher, and microwave. Some microwaves come with a braille overlay or large-print labels that can be ordered from the manufacturer. Microwaves with timer knobs may be the easiest to use and can be marked easily. Flat-panel microwaves can also be marked visually and tactilely to indicate the most common settings used.

Use of Color Contrast

As discussed in Lesson 1, use of color contrast is very effective in helping the resident with carrying out all sorts of tasks. The following recommendations are for use of color contrast in the food preparation area.

- Suggest the resident use plastic trays or cutting boards of contrasting colors on which to prepare foods. For example, cut a red apple on a white cutting board or place a dark mixing bowl on a white plastic tray or cutting board. Similarly, use a dark tray or cutting board for preparing a light-colored food, such as a potato.
- Tape a dark piece of paper to the wall to help improve visibility when pouring light liquids into a measuring cup. Hold up a measuring cup with dark liquids against a light piece of paper or a light-colored wall.

Preparing Simple Foods

Learning a few techniques for food preparation will help you in making suggestions to the residents. The following are some techniques for measuring.

TECHNIQUES FOR MEASURING

- Hold a light-colored measuring cup against a dark background to see light ingredients.
- Use dark-colored measuring cups to provide contrast when measuring light-colored ingredients such as flour and sugar.
- Use a measuring cup with raised numbers on the side or mark the cup tactilely with Hi-Marks.

- Use individual or stacked measuring cups to scoop the item to be measured. Some cups come with longer or bent handles for this task.
- Measure spices into the hand first to avoid pouring too much.
- For measuring wet ingredients, the resident may use the pouring techniques covered in Lesson 8 and use a finger or a liquid level indicator to know when to stop pouring.

Other food preparation techniques that you can teach residents are discussed in Lesson 8. These include

- pouring cold liquids
- pouring hot liquids
- adding salt and pepper
- spreading bread or toast with margarine, mayonnaise, or mustard

Useful Devices and Appliances

There are many useful kitchen devices and appliances available commercially and through the catalogs listed in Appendix B. Review these with the resident. Simple adaptations to existing kitchen equipment can be made to avoid large expenditures; however, some items that may be particularly useful include

- long oven mitts
- kitchen timer with raised markings or large print
- liquid-level indicator (see Lesson 8)
- safety food turner (double spatula)
- splatter shield
- cutting board with food chute for pouring
- cutting boards in light and dark colors to contrast with food
- color-coded or high-contrast measuring cups and spoons
- large-print and broad handle measuring cup
- adjustable knife with a slice guide for adjusting slices
- Hi-Marks for marking appliances

Congratulations! You have reached the end of Lesson 17. Now go on to the Key Points to review what you have learned in this lesson.

KEY POINTS IN LESSON 17

Safe Techniques for Preparing Foods

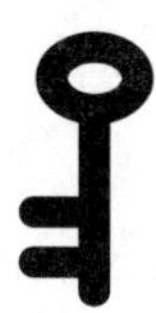

1. Review the task-lighting needs of the resident for kitchen work.
2. The principles of organization, labeling, and contrast are critical to enabling the resident with a visual impairment to prepare foods.
3. Mark appliances such as the stove dial with a substance such as Hi-Marks, which forms a raised marking when it dries, or another durable substance.
4. Various devices and appliances are available to help the resident with a visual impairment, such as marked measuring cups, liquid-level indicators, long oven gloves, and large-print and talking timers.

LEARNING ACTIVITIES

Try the following activities to practice what you have learned in this lesson. Some of the activities involve the use of simulators—glasses that simulate different types of vision loss. (See Appendix B for sources of vision simulators.) It is important to work in pairs while doing these exercises. One person uses the simulators while the other watches for safety and provides feedback.

- Using simulators, try to measure and pour several different substances.
- Using simulators, try to set the stove and/or microwave at a certain temperature, such as 350°F for the oven.
- Using simulators, try to identify a large-print label on a can.
- Review the types of devices and appliances available for use in the kitchen by older persons with visual impairments.

☑ SELF-CHECK

Indicate whether each statement is true (T) or false (F) in the space provided. Check Appendix A for the answers. Then go back and review any statements you may have missed.

______ 1. Many devices and appliances are available to help with tasks such as measuring, pouring, and cutting.

______ 2. Using Hi-Marks to mark a stove dial or other dials is a good technique.

LESSON 18 Sewing

GOAL

To show a resident who is visually impaired how to do routine sewing tasks.

OBJECTIVE

By the end of the lesson, you will be able to show the resident how to carry out routine sewing tasks.

TEACH Principles

As you review methods of sewing with the resident, use the five TEACH principles for working successfully with a resident who is visually impaired:

T—Talk to the resident about his or her sewing needs.

E—Encourage the resident to try out the sewing devices.

A—Assess the resident's interest in sewing.

C—"Can do" is the motto for each resident.

H—Help the resident to learn to use the sewing devices if he or she wishes to learn.

Continuing to Sew

Being able to maintain their clothes in good repair and do simple sewing tasks such as hemming helps residents continue to feel independent. Some residents may also enjoy needlecraft as a recreational activity.

Basic principles, such as the use of task lighting and color contrast, can help residents with sewing tasks. There are also a number of devices that can help residents who are visually impaired with sewing, especially with the sometimes difficult task of threading the needle.

General Hints for Sewing

USE OF TASK LIGHTING

As with other near tasks, such as reading and writing, task lighting—light shining directly on a task—can help the resident with a visual impairment to see a sewing project more distinctly. Review Lesson 9, Reading Techniques, for more tips on using task lighting.

USE OF COLOR CONTRAST

When possible, use color contrast when sewing. For example, place a light-colored fabric on a dark background while working. Using light thread with a dark fabric or vice versa will also help the resident see what he or she is sewing.

HELPFUL TOOLS

A variety of helpful tools or gadgets are available at most sewing stores.

- To help with hemming or sewing a straight line, use hem clips, which are available at most sewing stores. Safety pins can also be used.
- Use thread locks to keep the ends of threads from tangling.
- Liquid Stitch, a product that hardens when squeezed from a tube, can be used for hemming. This and similar products that

eliminate the need for at least some sewing are available at most sewing stores.

SEWING SAFETY

Dropped pins can be a safety hazard for residents. Use a magnet to locate dropped pins. Use it on the floor of the sewing area before vacuuming.

Threading Needles and Other Sewing Devices

Threading the needle can frequently be the most frustrating part of sewing for almost anyone. There are a number of devices that can help with this task. Regardless of how you thread the needle, it is always useful to place the point of the needle down into something that will stabilize it and help it stand up, such as a bar of soap, a piece of Styrofoam, or a cork.

NEEDLE THREADER

Thin metal needle threaders are commonly available for ordinary use. This small device has a loop made out of thin, flexible metal. The loop can be collapsed in order to fit through the eye of a needle. When it is pushed through the eye, it springs open into a loop again. It is then easy to pass the thread through the loop.

STEPS FOR USING A NEEDLE THREADER

STEP 1 Place the eye of the threader into the eye of the needle.

STEP 2 Pass the thread through the eye of the needle threader.

STEP 3 Pull the eye of the threader back out of the needle, and the needle is threaded.

STEP 4 Remove the thread from the needle threader.

SELF-THREADING NEEDLES

Self-threading needles are now available almost everywhere that sewing products are sold. They make it much easier for the person who is visually impaired to do mending or other sewing. In addition to a regular eye, the self-threading needle has a V-shaped opening in the top end, from which the thread can be pulled into the eye.

STEPS FOR USING SELF-THREADING NEEDLES

STEP 1 Stabilize the needle. Place the point of the needle into a bar of soap or a piece of Styrofoam, or a cork, to stabilize it.

STEP 2 Place the thread over needle. Place the thread over the center of the top of the needle.

STEP 3 Pull down so that the thread passes through the opening, allowing the needle to be threaded. You will hear or feel a slight click as this occurs.

PRELOADED NEEDLES

Some retail and sewing stores also have needles that are "preloaded"—already threaded—with thread available in several colors.

Congratulations! You have reached the end of Lesson 18. Now go on to the Key Points to review what you have learned in this lesson.

KEY POINTS IN LESSON 18

Sewing

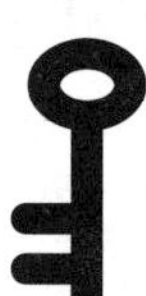

1. Be aware of basic principles such as use of color contrast and task lighting when helping residents sew.
2. Sewing devices such as self-threading needles and Liquid Stitch are available to assist with sewing.

LEARNING ACTIVITIES

Try the following activities to practice what you have learned in this lesson. Some of the activities involve the use of simulators—glasses that simulate different types of vision loss. (See Appendix B for sources of vision simulators.) It is important to work in pairs while doing these exercises. One person uses the simulators while the other watches for safety and provides feedback.

- Using simulators, practice threading a needle.
- Using simulators, practice sewing on a button.
- Teach another staff member to thread a needle.

☑ SELF-CHECK

Indicate whether each statement is true (T) or false (F) in the space provided. Check Appendix A for the answers. Then go back and review any statements you may have missed.

______ 1. Self-threading needles can help a resident who is unable to see to thread a needle.

______ 2. Placing the fabric on a contrasting surface can help a resident see what he or she is doing when sewing.

LESSON 19 Adaptive Games and Other Recreational Activities

GOAL

To know about recreational options for the older resident with a visual impairment.

OBJECTIVE

By the end of the lesson, you will be familiar with games and other recreational activities to suggest to the resident.

TEACH Principles

As you review recreational options with the resident, use the five TEACH principles for working successfully with a resident who is visually impaired:

T—**Talk** to the resident about games and exercises and explain them thoroughly

E—**Encourage** the resident to try using adaptive games.

A—**Assess** the resident's interest in participating in games.

C—"**Can do**" is the motto for each resident.

H—**Help** the resident to learn about recreational options.

Recreational Activities

Being involved in recreational activities is often important to residents with a visual impairment. They may feel, however, that due to their vision loss they can no longer participate in the activities they previously enjoyed or learn new ones.

Residents should be encouraged to continue to engage in activities that have always interested them, such as reading, bowling, golf, or attending concerts. You can assist them by telling them about adapted games and other ways of continuing their leisure activities. There are national associations for people who are blind or visually impaired that are devoted to particular sports, such as golf or bowling, that can provide more information about those activities. These are listed in Appendix B. Lesson 9 covers reading materials available in large print and tape.

Adapted Games

Many games are available commercially in an adapted format for people who are visually impaired—in versions with large print or tactile markings. Most of the following games are available through the catalogs listed in Appendix B.

- Checkers set with brightly contrasting colors for easy visibility. The white sections of the board are lower than the colored sections to provide a tactile way of differentiating the squares. There is also a pocket for the checkers to sit in. The checkers are red and black and are shaped differently. Magnetic checkers are also very effective in keeping the pieces in place on the board.
- Chess set with holes in the board for the chess pieces to fit in. The chess pieces are black and white and can be shaped differently or have tactile markings.
- Braille dominos with raised black dots on a white surface for high contrast. They come in various sizes. There are also large-size dominoes with indented dots.
- Brailled Monopoly with brailled dots and playing cards in braille and large print.

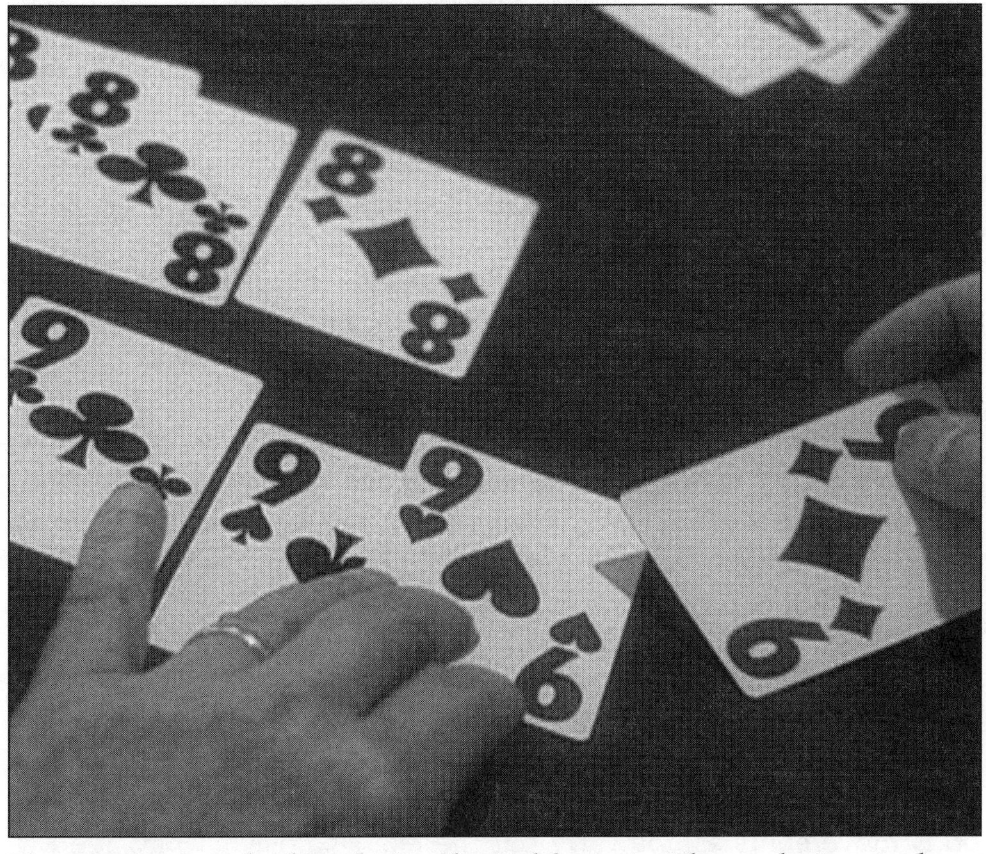

AMERICAN FOUNDATION FOR THE BLIND

Many games can be bought in adapted formats. These playing cards have large numbers and symbols in different colors.

- Low vision playing cards with 1.5-inch numbers and letters. Each suit has a different color. There are also brailled plastic playing cards so the braille won't wear out.
- Large-print and braille bingo cards that also have print
- Large-print crossword puzzles
- Braille dice

The basic principles mentioned in Lesson 1, such as using contrast and tactile indicators, also apply to playing board games.

- Place a game on a dark-colored surface, such as a plain dark tablecloth, to provide contrast with the edge of the board.
- Use markers or game pieces that contrast with the playing board; for example, you can use large poker chips as markers on a bingo card.
- Pieces that are tactilely different can be used for games such as Monopoly.

Adapting Fitness Exercises and Sports

Adaptive equipment for bowling and other types of sports is available. Contact the Blind Bowlers Association, and see catalogs in Appendix B for adapted equipment.

It is critical for older people to continue some type of physical activity. A recommendation from the Centers for Disease Control and Prevention states, "Every adult should accumulate 30 minutes or more of moderate physical activity over most days of the week." This recommendation applies to older people with disabilities, including those with visual impairment (of course, the resident's doctor should be consulted before embarking on new physical activities). Moderate activity can include walking, gardening, exercise class, dancing, or any type of physical movement.

If the resident chooses to take an exercise class, take care to explain the exercise in detail. Remember that the more verbal cues you can give a resident who is visually impaired, the better the resident will be able to understand how to do the exercise. When instructing the resident, you may need to allow him or her to feel your body movements as you carry out the exercise or you may need to place a resident's arm in a proper position to do the exercise. Always ask the resident before touching him or her and explain what you need to do.

Also, be aware that visually impaired persons may have balance problems and may need to use a sturdy chair, another person, or a cane to balance themselves.

WATCHING TELEVISION

Some residents prefer to use small television sets so that they can see the screen by sitting closely. Others prefer a large screen, which they may be able to see from a short distance.

Some residents may be able to see black-and-white TV better than color, whereas others will see color better.

Watch out for glare from a window or mirror when positioning the TV (see Lesson 4). If sunlight or a lamp is shining directly on the screen, it will produce glare. Try to position the TV with the sun or light behind it. The best option is to position the TV on a blank wall, if possible. Turning on a light in the room sometimes helps the resident with watching TV, as long as the light does not reflect on the screen or cause glare.

Some television programs and films on videotape are available with descriptions of what is being shown on the screen inserted on the sound track. This is called *video description*. See Appendix B for more information on how to get video-described programs.

You can mark the remote tactilely to help residents with its use. Sometimes placing a rubber band under the center row of numbers, 4,5,6, helps the resident with tactile orientation to the numbers.

If the resident uses a remote, he or she should designate a specific place to keep it so it is easy to locate.

Encouragement

When you talk to older residents about recreational activities, remember the "E" of the TEACH principles: Encourage. An older resident may have recently lost vision and feel unable to continue former activities. You will need to help build the resident's self-esteem and self-confidence. A local support group of individuals with visual impairments may be available to help.

Congratulations! You have reached the end of Lesson 19. Now go on to the Key Points to review what you have learned in this lesson.

KEY POINTS IN LESSON 19

Adaptive Games and Other Recreational Activities

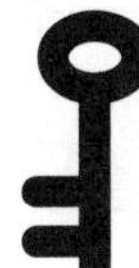

1. Many games have been adapted for use by persons who are visually impaired. Some include
   - checkers
   - cards
   - bingo
   - chess
2. Residents who are visually impaired can engage in most exercises that others perform—depending, of course, on their physical and mental capabilities. When helping a resident, do the following:
   - Explain how to perform the exercise.
   - Demonstrate, letting the resident feel how you do it.
   - Be aware that visually impaired persons may have balance problems.

LEARNING ACTIVITIES

Try the following activities to practice what you have learned in this lesson. Some of the activities involve the use of simulators—glasses that simulate different types of vision loss. (See Appendix B for sources of vision simulators.) It is important to work in pairs while doing these exercises. One person uses the simulators while the other watches for safety and provides feedback.

- Using the simulators, try playing a game that has been adapted.
- Try to explain how to play a game to another staff member who is wearing simulators.
- Familiarize yourself with types of adapted games that are available.

SELF-CHECK

Indicate whether each statement is true (T) or false (F) in the space provided. Check Appendix A for the answers. Then go back and review any statements you may have missed.

______ 1. Residents who are visually impaired should give up watching TV, since they can't see it very well.

______ 2. Residents who are visually impaired can play bingo or card games if given the right equipment and instruction.

LESSON 20 Shopping

GOAL

To assist the resident with a visual impairment to continue or resume shopping.

OBJECTIVES

By the end of the lesson, you will be able to

- ➤ provide information and guidance about shopping to the resident
- ➤ make suggestions to the management of a store about making the store an easier place to shop

TEACH Principles

As you review information about shopping with the resident, use the five TEACH principles for working successfully with a resident who is visually impaired:

T—Talk to the resident about shopping.

E—Encourage the resident to try shopping if appropriate.

A—Assess the resident's ability to shop, including any other limitations besides visual impairment.

C—"Can do" is the motto for each resident.

H—Help the resident to learn techniques about shopping with a visual impairment if he or she wishes to learn.

Concerns about Stores

This lesson applies to residents who are able to go out shopping. Shopping may have been an important activity for a resident before becoming visually impaired. Being able to continue to provide the necessities of daily life is important to a resident's self-esteem.

Stores, however, are often not user-friendly for consumers with visual impairments. Glare in the store from large, unshaded windows and the type of flooring used can make it difficult to navigate the store and find items. Often, some aisles are brightly lighted, whereas others are too dim. Signs may be difficult to read.

Shopping Solutions

There are a number of ways you can help residents with shopping. You can address environmental issues in the store, help the resident get assistance while shopping, and show the resident helpful techniques for shopping.

STORE ENVIRONMENT

You can talk to the store manager about some of the glare and lighting problems. Other customers may be experiencing similar problems and the manager may not be aware of the situation. The manager may be able to make a few changes, such as reducing glare from windows and floors, using spot lighting in darker areas, and using signs that are easier to read. In the long run, these changes will make the store safer and more accessible to anyone experiencing normal vision changes related to aging.

In addition, if overhead glare in the store continues to be a problem, suggest the resident try wearing a sun visor while shopping.

ASKING FOR ASSISTANCE

If the resident is unable to find items independently, suggest the resident ask for help from the management to assign a clerk to provide assistance. If the resident feels uncomfortable, help the resident practice asking for help. Introduce the resident to the manager.

Some stores offer a shopper assistance service. The resident may need to call ahead to see what services are available.

SHOPPING TECHNIQUES

There are a number of techniques that can help residents with visual impairments find their way around and identify items while shopping.

- First, orient the resident to the store. Take the resident around to each department, helping to find the locations of items the resident usually buys.
- Encourage the resident to use a magnifier to pick out favorite brands and read the labels.
- For shopping in a grocery store, encourage the resident to use other senses besides vision to pick out items. By smelling and feeling produce, for example, you can identify foods and select items of good quality. You can also shake cans and use touch and hearing to help identify the contents. For instance, a can of corn will slosh around when shaken but cream corn will not. This technique can help when labels look the same and reading the label is too difficult.

Congratulations! You have reached the end of Lesson 20. Now go on to the Key Points to review what you have learned in this lesson.

KEY POINTS IN LESSON 20

Shopping

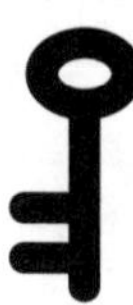

1. Grocery stores, department stores, and smaller shops are often not user-friendly for people who are visually impaired.
2. Some changes that can be made to make shopping easier for a resident include
   - glare control
   - use of contrast
   - better lighting in specific areas of the store
   - clearer signs
   - awareness of visual impairment on the part of management and store clerks
3. Residents may need to be oriented to the store and where certain items are kept.
4. Residents may need assistance in locating items and may need to practice soliciting help.

LEARNING ACTIVITIES

Try the following activities to practice what you have learned in this lesson. Some of the activities involve the use of simulators—glasses that simulate different types of vision loss. (See Appendix B for sources of vision simulators.) It is important to work in pairs while doing these exercises. One person uses the simulators while the other watches for safety and provides feedback.

- Go to your favorite grocery or other type of store and put on a set of simulators.
- Walk around the store, making notes about ways in which to make the store a more accessible place to shop for residents with visual impairments.

☑ SELF-CHECK

Indicate whether each statement is true (T) or false (F) in the space provided. Check Appendix A for the answers. Then go back and review any statements you may have missed.

______ 1. The store manager needs to be made aware of things he or she can do to make the store more accessible for individuals with visual impairments.

______ 2. Residents should be taught to solicit aid in a grocery store when they are unable to find grocery items or read the labels.

Posttest on Age-Related Vision Loss

Congratulations on completing the curriculum! Now, take a moment to assess what you have learned by completing the following posttest. Indicate whether the statement is true (T) or false (F) in the space provided. The answers to the test can be found in Appendix A.

______ 1. Normal changes in the eye as people grow older include need for more light, presbyopia, and myopia.

______ 2. There are two types of visual field loss resulting from various eye conditions—central vision loss and side vision loss.

______ 3. The major eye diseases associated with aging are cataracts, macular degeneration, glaucoma, and diabetic retinopathy.

______ 4. Vision loss can be caused by stroke.

______ 5. Evaluating the resident's environment for glare, lighting, and contrast is a key strategy to help the older resident function more independently.

______ 6. Sighted guide is used to teach guide dogs to work with individuals who are blind.

______ 7. Most people who experience age-related vision loss become totally blind.

______ 8. A resident who is experiencing sudden hazy or blurred vision, double vision, or recurring pain in or around the eyes should be checked as soon as possible by an eye care specialist.

______ 9. Loss of side vision can make doing tasks such as reading difficult for the resident.

______ 10. Writing is an activity that an older person with age-related vision loss has to give up.

APPENDIX A

Answer Key to True/False Questions

INTRODUCTION: PRETEST ON AGING-RELATED VISION LOSS
1. F; 2. F; 3. T; 4. T; 5. T; 6. F; 7. F; 8. T; 9. F; 10. F

LESSON 1 1. T; 2. T; 3. T

LESSON 2 1. F; 2. F; 3.T

LESSON 3 1. T; 2. F; 3. F; 4. T

LESSON 4 1. F; 2. T; 3. F

LESSON 5 1. F; 2. F; 3. T

LESSON 6 1. T; 2. T; 3. T; 4. T

LESSON 7 1. T; 2. T

LESSON 8 1. F; 2. T; 3. T

LESSON 9 1. T; 2. T; 3. T

LESSON 10 1. T; 2. T

LESSON 11 1. T; 2. F

LESSON 12 1. T; 2. T

LESSON 13 1. T; 2. F

LESSON 14 1. F; 2. T

LESSON 15 1. T; 2. T

LESSON 16 1. T; 2. T

LESSON 17 1. T; 2. T

LESSON 18 1. T; 2. T

LESSON 19 1. F; 2. T

LESSON 20 1. T; 2. T

POSTTEST ON AGING-RELATED VISION LOSS
1. F; 2. F; 3. T; 4. T; 5. T; 6.F; 7. F; 8. T; 9. F; 10. F

APPENDIX B

Resources

This resource listing provides a sample of the organizations and companies that offer assistance, information, referrals, products, and services related to vision loss and aging. If these organizations and companies do not have the answers to questions regarding residents with vision loss, they will be able to refer you to someplace that does.

For ease of use, this appendix is divided into a few main sections: sources of information and referrals; sources of vision simulators; sources of all kinds of products for independent living; and resources for recreation.

For more complete listings of resources, you can consult the AFB *Directory of Services for Blind and Visually Impaired Persons in the United States and Canada*, available from the American Foundation for the Blind or online at www.afb.org.

Information and Referral

The organizations listed in this section provide general information about visual impairment and blindness, eye conditions, and adapted or specialized products and technology, as well as referrals for additional information and services.

GENERAL INFORMATION ON VISUAL IMPAIRMENT

AMERICAN ACADEMY OF OPHTHALMOLOGY
P.O. Box 7424
San Francisco, CA 94120
www.eyenet.org
(415) 561-8500
Fax: (415) 561-8533
E-mail: comm@aao.org

The professional membership association for eye care physicians, works to ensure that the public can obtain the best possible eye care. Provides information on eye health for consumers and referrals to member physicians.

AMERICAN FOUNDATION FOR THE BLIND
11 Penn Plaza, Suite 300
New York, NY 10001
www.afb.org
(800) 232-5463 (800-AFB-LINE) or (212) 502-7600
Fax: (212) 502-7777
E-mail: afbinfo@afb.net

Provides services to and acts as an information clearinghouse for people who are blind or visually impaired and their families, professionals, organizations, schools, and corporations. Has fact sheets on many aspects of visual impairment, including aging and vision loss. Stimulates research and mounts program initiatives to improve services to blind and visually impaired people. Publishes a wide variety of professional, reference, and consumer books and videos; journals; and the AFB *Directory of Services for Blind and Visually Impaired Persons in the United States and Canada*.

AMERICAN OPTOMETRIC ASSOCIATION
243 North Lindbergh Boulevard
St. Louis, MO 63141
www.aoanet.org
(314) 991-4100
Fax: (314) 991-4101

Provides information on visual conditions, eye diseases, and low vision; consumer guides for eye care; and referrals to optometrists.

HADLEY SCHOOL FOR THE BLIND
700 Elm Street
Winnetka, IL 60093-0299
www.hadley-school.org
(800) 323-4238
Fax: (847) 446-0855
E-mail: info@Hadley-School.org

Offers tuition-free distance education courses for persons who are legally blind, their family members, and professionals and paraprofessionals working in the blindness field. Courses include Conducting Self-Help Groups; You, Your Eyes, and Your Diabetes; Self-Esteem and Adjusting with Blindness; Introduction to Low Vision; Independent Living; Recreation and Leisure Time Activities. Also offers high school courses, as well as courses in braille and communication skills, independent living, recreation and leisure, and technology.

HELEN KELLER NATIONAL CENTER FOR DEAF-BLIND YOUTHS AND ADULTS
111 Middle Neck Road
Sands Point, NY 11050-1299
www.helenkeller.org
(516) 944-8900
Fax: (516) 944-7302

TDD/TTY: (516) 944-8637
E-mail: hknctrng@aol.com

Works to assist persons with deaf-blindness in becoming as independent as possible and in enjoying a quality of life as full and productive as possible. Has an aging specialist as well.

LIGHTHOUSE INTERNATIONAL
111 East 59th Street
New York, NY 10022-1202
www.lighthouse.org
(800) 829-0500, (888) 222-9320, or (212) 821-9200
(consumer referral line)
TTY: (212) 821-9713
E-mail: info@lighthouse.org

Works to overcome visual impairment for people of all ages through worldwide leadership in rehabilitation services, education, research, and advocacy. Provides rehabilitation services, including training in adaptive living skills and computer skills for seniors. Publishes *Aging & Vision* newsletter and other publications on age-related vision loss for both professional and lay audiences. Maintains a catalog of independent living products.

NATIONAL ASSOCIATION FOR VISUALLY HANDICAPPED
22 West 21st Street
New York, NY 10010
www.navh.org
(212) 889-3141
Fax: (212) 727-2931
E-mail: staff@navh.org
or 3201 Balboa Street
San Francisco, CA 94121
(415) 221-3201
Fax: (415) 221-8754
E-mail: staffca@navh.org

Provides information and referral for people with low vision on large-print books, low vision devices, medical advances and updates, craft materials and projects, resource guides, and religious materials. Sells low vision products and devices. Maintains a large-print mail-order library. Promotes public awareness of low vision.

NATIONAL EYE CARE PROJECT
P.O. Box 429098
San Francisco, CA 94142-9098
www.eyenet.org
(800) 222-3937 or (887) 888-6327
Fax: (415) 561-8567

Provides medical and surgical eye care for persons over 65 years of age at no out-of-pocket cost through a network of volunteer ophthalmologists around the country. Provides literature on eye diseases and procedures.

U.S. DEPARTMENT OF VETERANS AFFAIRS BLIND REHABILITATION SERVICE
810 Vermont Avenue, NW
Washington, DC 20420
www.va.gov/blindrehab/index.cfm
(888) 442-4551 or (202) 273-8481
Fax: (202) 273-7603

Oversees programs for visually impaired veterans through a network of rehabilitation centers, clinics, and field staff throughout the country. Services include orientation and mobility, living skills, communication skills, activities of daily living, manual skills, computer access training, physical conditioning, recreation, adjustment to blindness, family counseling, and group meetings. Also supplies needed aids and appliances and equipment.

SPECIFIC EYE CONDITIONS

AMERICAN DIABETES ASSOCIATION
1701 North Beauregard Street
Alexandria, VA 22314
www.diabetes.org
(703) 549-1500 (local),
(800) 342-2383, (888) 342-2383,
or (888) DIABETES
(for referral to local offices)
Fax: (703) 549-6995 E-mail:
customerservice@diabetes.org

Provides information and public education about diabetes, including diabetic retinopathy, to consumers and professionals. Publishes books, journals, and brochures.

AMERICAN MACULAR DEGENERATION FOUNDATION
P.O. Box 515
Northampton, MA 01061-0515
www.macular.org
(413) 268-7660

Works for the prevention, treatment, and cure of macular degeneration by raising funds, educating the public, and supporting scientific research. Provides consumer information and referrals to eye care professionals.

AMERICAN SOCIETY OF CATARACT AND REFRACTIVE SURGERY
4000 Legato Road, Suite 850
Fairfax, VA 22033
www.ascrs.org
(703) 591-2220 Fax: (703) 591-0614
E-mail: ascrs@ascrs.org

Provides information about cataracts and cataract and refractive surgery and referrals to ophthalmologists specializing in eye surgery.

GLAUCOMA FOUNDATION
116 John Street, Suite 1605
New York, NY 10038
www.glaucoma-foundation.org
(212) 285-0080 or (800) GLAUCOMA
(800-452-8266) E-mail:
info@glaucoma-foundation.org

Offers information and public education about glaucoma; provides free glaucoma screenings; funds research; and publishes consumer guides and brochures and *Eye to Eye*, a quarterly newsletter.

Sources of Vision Simulators

The following organizations and companies distribute vision simulators—glasses that simulate different types of functional vision loss. They can be used for the learning activities in this training manual. The type and cost of the simulators vary among distributors.

ASSOCIATION FOR EDUCATION AND REHABILITATION OF THE BLIND AND VISUALLY IMPAIRED (AER) DIVISION 7 (LOW VISION)
c/o Marshall Flax
754 Williamson Street
Madison, WI 53703-3115
(608) 255-6178
Fax: (608) 255-3301
E-mail: Marshall@wcblind.org

Supplies a variety of simulators showing different degrees of various eye conditions, including age-related macular degeneration, retinitis pigmentosa, glaucoma, diabetic retinopathy, and cataracts.

DAAS CONSULTING
P.O. Box 93545
Nelson Park PO
Vancouver, BC V6E 4L7
Canada
E-mail: daascon@istar.ca

Distributes vision problem simulation kits for professionals.

LIGHTHOUSE INTERNATIONAL
111 East 59th Street
New York, NY 10022
www.lighthouse.org
(800) 334-5497 or (212) 821-9200
TDD: (212) 821-9713
E-mail: info@lighthouse.org

Sells VisualEyes Simulators, a set of disposable glasses that simulate functional vision loss.

DR. GEORGE ZIMMERMAN
Program Coordinator
University of Pittsburgh
School of Education
Department of Instruction and Learning
4H01 Forbes Quadrangle
Pittsburgh, PA 15260
www:pitt.edu/~soeforum/sped_vis.html
(412) 624-7254
Fax: (412) 648-7081

Sells vision simulators.

Products for Independent Living

GENERAL INDEPENDENT LIVING CATALOGS

The companies listed in this section sell by catalog a wide variety of specialized products that help people with visual impairments and other disabilities carry out everyday activities. The types of products in each catalog are indicated in the listing.

ABLEWARE/MADDAK
www.maddak.com
(973) 628-7600
Fax: (973) 305-0841
E-mail: custservice@maddak.com

Designer and manufacturer of assistive devices for activities of daily living. Offers adapted games, adapted scissors, eating utensils and tableware, enlarged grips, nonskid table mats, and writing devices.

AMERICAN PRINTING HOUSE FOR THE BLIND
1839 Frankfort Avenue
P.O. Box 6085
Louisville, KY 40206-0085
www.aph.org
(502) 895-2405 or (800) 223-1839
Fax: (502) 899-2274
E-mail: catalogs@aph.org (request a catalog)
or cs@aph.org (customer service)

The Adult Life Products catalog features braille products, books, and supplies; large-print books; computer software and access products; labeling and marking products; lighting; low vision devices; mobility devices; personal care products; recreation and leisure products; talking products; and writing and reading devices.

ANN MORRIS ENTERPRISES
551 Hosner Mountain Road
Stormville, NY 12582
www.annmorris.com
(800) 454-3175 or (845) 227-9659
Fax: (845) 226-2793

Braille products and supplies, adapted clocks and watches, computer software and access products, diabetes management products, kitchen and housekeeping items, labeling and marking products, lighting, low vision devices, mobility devices, personal care products, recreation and leisure products, talking products, telephones and accessories, and writing and reading devices.

CLOTILDE
Box 3000
Louisiana, MO 63353-3000
www.clotilde.com
(800) 545-5002
E-mail: webmaster@clotilde.com

Sewing notions, needle threaders, and regular and adaptive sewing supplies.

INDEPENDENT LIVING AIDS
200 Robbins Lane
Jericho, NY 11753
www.independentliving.com
(800) 537-2118 or (516) 937-1848
Fax: (516) 937-3906
E-mail:
can-do@independentliving.com

Braille products and supplies, adapted clocks and watches, computer software and access products, diabetes management products, kitchen and housekeeping items, labeling and marking products, lighting, low vision devices, mobility devices, personal care products, recreation and leisure products, talking products, telephones and accessories, and writing and reading devices.

THE LIGHTHOUSE CATALOG
111 East 59th Street
New York, NY 10022-1202
www.lighthouse.org and
www.thelighthousecatalog.com
(888) 770-7660

Adapted clocks and watches, diabetes management products, kitchen and housekeeping items, labeling and marking products, lighting, low vision devices, mobility devices, personal care products, recreation and leisure products, talking products, telephones and accessories, and writing and reading devices.

LS&S GROUP
P.O. Box 673
Northbrook, IL 60065
(800) 468-4789
TDD: (800) 317-8583
Fax: (847) 498-1482
E-mail: lssgrp@aol.com

Braille products and supplies, adapted clocks and watches, computer software and access products, diabetes management products, kitchen and housekeeping items, labeling and marking products, lighting, low vision devices, mobility devices, personal care products, recreation and leisure products, talking products, telephones and accessories, and writing and reading devices.

MAXI-AIDS
42 Executive Boulevard
Farmingdale, NY 11735
www.maxiaids.com
(800) 522-6294 (orders) and (631) 752-0521 (information)
TTY: (631) 752-0738
Fax: (631) 752-0689
E-mail: sales@maxiaids.com

Braille products and supplies, adapted clocks and watches, computer software and access products, diabetes management products, kitchen and housekeeping items, labeling and marking products, lighting, low vision devices, mobility devices, personal care products, recreation and leisure products, talking products, telephones and accessories, and writing and reading devices.

LIGHTING PRODUCTS

The companies listed here specialize in products that can help improve the lighting in your facility. See also the previous section, General Independent Living Catalogs, for other sources of lighting, lamps, and lightbulbs.

A.L.P. LIGHTING COMPONENTS
6333 Gross Point Road
Niles, IL, 60714-3915
www.alp-ltg.com
(773) 774-9550
Fax: (773) 774-9331
E-mail: info@alp-ltg.com

Manufacturer of a wide variety of lighting fixtures, lamps, lightbulbs, louvers, reflectors, and compact fluorescent bulbs.

DAZOR MANUFACTURING CORPORATION
4483 Duncan Avenue
St Louis, MO 63110
www.dazor.com
(800) 345-9103 or (314) 652-2400
Fax: (314) 652-2069
E-mail: info@dazor.com

Manufacturer of a wide variety of task lights and lamps, including swing arm, combination fluorescent/incandescent, halogen, and magnifying.

PHILIPS LIGHTING COMPANY
200 Franklin Square Drive
Somerset, NJ 08875-6800
www.lighting.philips.com
(800) 555-0050 or (732) 563-1731
Fax: (732) 563-3740

Manufacturer of a wide variety of lightbulbs, including fluorescent, compact fluorescent, incandescent, halogen, and full spectrum. Also provides specialty lighting and innovative lighting solutions.

PRODUCTS FOR LABELING

The companies listed here specialize in products for labeling and identification. See the section General Independent Living Catalogs in this appendix for other sources of products for labeling and marking, including clothing identifiers, Hi-Marks 3-D Marker, Spot 'n Line Pen, prescription labels, raised marks and dots, and marking pens and materials.

Talking Prescription Labels

EN-VISION AMERICA
1013 Porter Lane
Normal, IL 61761
www.envisionamerica.com
(800) 890-1180 or (309) 452-3088
Fax: (309) 452-3643
E-mail:
envision@envisionamerica.com

Distributors of ScripTalk, a portable, handheld audio system, which reads prescriptions aloud.

RX PARTNERS PHARMACY
500 Old Pond Road, Suite 403
Bridgeville, PA 15017
www.rxpartnerspharmacy.com
(888) 477-6337

Distributor of Aloud, an audio system that reads prescription labels aloud.

MILLENNIUM COMPLIANCE CORPORATION
P.O. Box 649
Southington, CT 06489
www.talkingrx.com
(860) 426-0542

Distributor of Talking Rx, an audio system that reads prescription label aloud.

Marking, Labeling, and Identification Products

GLADYS E. LOEB FOUNDATION
2002 Forest Hill Drive
Silver Spring, MD 20903-1532
(301) 434-7748 (telephone or fax)

Manufacturer of Loeb's Labels, durable plastic nonbraille food labels in the shapes of popular fruits and vegetables, mounted on durable elastic bands.

SETON IDENTIFICATION PRODUCTS
Department AR-11
20 Thompson Road
P.O. Box 819
Branford, CT 06405-0819
www.seton.com
(800) 243-6624

Safety signs, safety labels, sign and label machines, reflective tape, warning tape, marking materials, and large-print letters.

Resources for Recreation

READING

The sources listed here provide reading materials in alternate formats, including large-print, braille, or audio. See also the section General Independent Living Catalogs in this appendix for products that can help with reading, such as closed-circuit television systems, computer adaptations, computer hardware and software, and additional large-print reading materials, including cookbooks.

CHOICE MAGAZINE LISTENING
P.O. Box 10
Port Washington, NY 11050
(516) 883-8280
Fax: (516) 944-6849

A free monthly anthology of current articles chosen from over 100 leading magazines. Recorded in four-track Library of Congress format. Distributed free through regional libraries. Also available through individual subscription.

CIL PUBLICATIONS AND AUDIOBOOKS
500 Greenwich Street, 3rd floor
New York, NY 10013
www.cilpubs.com
(888) CIL-8333
Fax: (212) 219-4078
E-mail: cilpubs@visionsvcb.org

Offers self-study audiotapes and audiobooks for people who are blind or visually impaired. Subjects include indoor mobility, personal management, and sensory development.

DOUBLEDAY LARGE PRINT HOME LIBRARY
6550 East 30th Street
P.O. Box 6309
Indianapolis, IN 46206-6309
(371) 541-8920

Offers a large-print Book-of-the-Month Club.

INTERNATIONAL ASSOCIATION OF AUDIO INFORMATION SERVICES
http://iaais.org
(800) 280-5325

An international organization of radio reading services that provides audio access to information for people who are print disabled (blind, visually impaired, learning disabled, or physically disabled), including news, feature stories, sports, advertisements, and other special programs. Connects listeners with services in their area.

IN TOUCH NETWORKS
15 West 65th Street
New York, NY 10023
(212) 769-6270

Provides national programming services for local radio reading services for people who are blind or visually impaired. Offers closed-circuit radio broadcasts of national and local newspapers and magazines.

MATILDA ZIEGLER MAGAZINE FOR THE BLIND
20 West 17th Street
New York, NY 10011
(212) 242-0263

Publishes the *Matilda Ziegler Magazine for the Blind*, a free monthly general-interest periodical. Provided in braille and on audiocassette.

NATIONAL LIBRARY SERVICE FOR THE BLIND AND PHYSICALLY HANDICAPPED
Library of Congress
1291 Taylor Street, NW
Washington, DC 20011
http://lcweb.loc.gov/nls
(202) 707-5100 or (800) 424-8567
TDD: (202) 707-0744
Fax: (202) 707-0712
E-mail: nls@loc.gov

Provides a free library service for people who are unable to read standard print materials because of a visual or physical impairment. Recorded Talking Books and magazines and braille publications are delivered to eligible borrowers by postage-free mail and through a network of cooperative libraries. Also distributes Talking Book machines.

NEW YORK TIMES LARGE-TYPE WEEKLY
229 West 43rd Street
New York, NY 10036
www.nytimes.com
(800) 631-2580
(information and subscriptions)

Publishes a weekly news summary from the *New York Times*.

READER'S DIGEST FUND FOR THE BLIND
P.O. Box 241
Mount Morris, IL 61054
www.readersdigest.com
800-877-5293
(information and subscriptions)

Offers selections from *Reader's Digest*, Reader's Digest condensed books, and other Reader's Digest publications.

VIDEO DESCRIPTION

Some television programs and films on videotape are available in video-described versions; that is, they have explanations and descriptions of the visual elements inserted on the sound track without interfering with the sounds and dialogue that are part of the program. For some television programs, these descriptions can be heard on a separate audio channel that is available on most stereo televisions sold in the United States. This channel is called Secondary Audio Program, or SAP. Programs are available on many public broadcasting and cable stations, and video-described movies can be purchased or borrowed from some libraries and video stores.

DESCRIPTIVE VIDEO SERVICE: MEDIA ACCESS GROUP AT WGBH
125 Western Avenue
Boston, MA 02134
www.wgbh.org/access
(617) 300-3600 (local) or
(800) 333-1203 (prerecorded information only)
Fax: (617) 300-1020
E-mail: access@wgbh.org

NARRATIVE TELEVISION NETWORK (NTN)
5840 South Memorial Drive, Suite 312
Tulsa, OK 74145-9082
www.narrativetv.com
(918) 627-1000 or (800) 801-8184
Fax: (918) 627-4101 E-mail: webmaster@narrativetv.com

OTHER RECREATIONAL OPPORTUNITIES

The organizations listed here provide information on just a few of the many recreational opportunities available to people who are blind or visually impaired.

AMERICAN BLIND BOWLING ASSOCIATION
315 North Main
Houston, PA 15342
(724) 745-5986

Promotes bowling for people who are blind or visually impaired. Administers leagues and sponsors tournaments.

UNITED STATES BLIND GOLF ASSOCIATION
304 Shamrock Street North
Tallahassee, FL 32308
www.blindgolf.com
(850) 893-4511
E-mail: usbga@blindgolf.com

Provides opportunities for golfers who are blind or visually impaired to compete with their peers.

APPENDIX C

Tips for Print Readability

Impaired vision may make reading difficult because of one or more of the following factors:

- a reduced amount of light entering the eye
- a blurred image on the retina
- a defective macula (the central portion of the retina), which is needed for reading

Reduced light and blurring affects the contrast of the print against its background. Damage to the central retina interferes with the ability to see small print and to make the eye movements necessary for reading.

The following are guidelines to making print more legible for individuals with these vision problems. However, these tips will make reading easier not only for individuals with low vision but for the general public as well.

PRINT SIZE

Large-print type should be used, preferably print in 18 point, but at least in 16 point. Scaleable fonts on the computer make this easy to do.

FONT TYPE AND STYLE

The goal in font selection is to use easily recognizable characters, either standard roman or sans serif fonts.

- Avoid decorative fonts.
- Use bold type because the thickness of the letters makes the print more legible.
- Avoid using italics or all capital letters. Both these forms of print make it more difficult to differentiate among letters.

COLOR

The use of different-colored letters for headings and emphasis is difficult to read for many people with low vision. When color is used, dark blues and greens are most effective.

CONTRAST

Contrast is one of the most critical factors in enhancing visual functioning, for printed materials as well as in environmental design. Text should be printed with the best possible contrast. For many older people, light lettering—either white or light-yellow—on a dark background, usually black, is easier to read than black lettering on a white or ivory background.

PAPER QUALITY

Avoid using glossy-finish paper such as that typically used in magazines and some journals. Glossy pages create excess glare, which increases reading difficulty for people who have low vision.

LEADING (SPACE BETWEEN LINES OF TEXT)

The recommended spacing between lines of text should be 1.5, rather than single space. Many people who are visually impaired have difficulty finding the beginning of the next line when single spacing is used.

TRACKING (SPACING BETWEEN LETTERS)

Text with letters very close together makes reading difficult for many people who are visually impaired, particularly for those who have central visual field defects, such as older persons with macular degeneration. Spacing between letters should be wide, such as that in monospaced fonts—fonts that have an equal amount of space allocated for each letter—such as Courier.

MARGINS

Many low vision devices, such as stand magnifiers and closed circuit televisions (CCTVs), are easiest to use on a flat surface. When material is bound or placed in a binder, an extra-wide margin in the center makes it easier to hold the material flat. A minimum of one inch should be used; one and a half inches is preferable.

Research is still under way to determine ways of making text more legible for individuals with limited vision.

APPENDIX D

How to Recognize Vision Loss in Older People

There are certain behaviors that indicate an individual may be experiencing vision loss. Be alert if a person has difficulty in the following areas.

PERFORMING DAILY ACTIVITIES

- Changes the way that he or she reads, watches television, drives, walks, or performs hobbies. Or, he or she stops doing one or more of these activities.
- Squints or tilts the head to the side to get an object into focus.
- Has difficulty identifying faces or objects.
- Has difficulty locating personal objects, even in a familiar environment.
- Reaches out for objects in an uncertain manner.
- Has difficulty identifying colors and selects clothing in unusual color combinations.

READING AND WRITING

- Is no longer able read the mail or a newspaper.
- Holds reading material very close to the face or at an angle.

- Writes less clearly or precisely and has difficulty writing on the line.
- Finds lighting in the room inadequate for reading and other activities and requests additional lighting.

MOVING

- Brushes against the wall while walking.
- Consistently bumps into objects.
- Has difficulty walking on irregular or bumpy surfaces.
- Goes up and down stairs slowly and cautiously, even though he or she has no other physical limitations.

EATING AND DRINKING

- Has difficulty getting food onto a fork.
- Has difficulty cutting food or serving himself or herself from a serving plate.
- Spills food off the plate while eating.
- Pours liquids over the top of the cup.
- Knocks over liquids while reaching across the table for another item.

If you notice any of these behaviors, encourage the older person to have an eye examination by an eye care specialist, either an ophthalmologist or optometrist, and a low vision evaluation by a low vision specialist, usually an optometrist or ophthalmologist with a specialization in low vision. Even if you do not notice these behaviors, it's important to encourage every older person to have an annual dilated eye examination.

APPENDIX E

Creating a Functional Environment for Older People Who Are Visually Impaired

The use of lighting and color contrast, and the reduction of glare, are important factors to be aware of in creating the best environment for older persons in general. They are crucial for older people with visual impairments. People working in the field of aging should take these factors into consideration when designing environments for all older persons, particularly in senior centers, retirement communities, assisted living environments, and nursing homes.

The suggestions that follow can be used to make an initial assessment of the environment. They include the primary environmental elements needed for older persons who are blind or visually impaired to be able to function independently in any environment. A vision rehabilitation professional can provide further assistance in assessing the environment and making recommendations for changes to enhance safe and independent functioning, and active participation, for older people with visual impairments.

LIGHTING

- In recreation and reading areas, provide plenty of floor lamps and table lamps.
- Advise people who are visually impaired that light should always be aimed at the work they are doing, not at the eyes.

- Replace burned-out lightbulbs regularly.
- Place mirrors so that lighting doesn't reflect off them and create glare.
- For window coverings, use adjustable blinds, sheer curtains, or draperies, because they allow for the adjustment of natural light.
- Keep a few chairs near windows for reading or doing handcrafts in natural light.

FURNITURE

- Arrange furniture in small groupings so that people can converse easily. Do not move furniture from place to place without informing people who are visually impaired.
- Make sure there is adequate lighting near furniture.
- When purchasing new furniture, select upholstery with texture when possible. Texture provides tactile clues for identification.
- Use brightly colored accessories, such as vases and lamps, to make furniture easier to locate.
- Avoid upholstery and floor coverings with patterns. Stripes and checks can create confusion for people who are visually impaired.

ELIMINATION OF HAZARDS

- Replace worn carpeting and floor coverings.
- Tape down or remove area rugs.
- Remove electrical cords from pathways, or tape down for safety.
- Do not wax floors; use nonskid, nonglare products to clean and polish floors.
- Keep desk chairs and table chairs pushed in.
- Move large pieces of furniture out of the main traffic areas.
- If telephone booths protrude into main traffic areas, have them moved.

USE OF COLOR CONTRAST

- Place light objects against a dark background—a dark table near a white wall, for example, or a black switch plate on a white wall.
- Install doorknobs that contrast in color with doors for easy location.
- Paint the woodwork of the door frame a contrasting color to make it easier to locate.
- Mark the edges of all steps and ramps with paint or tape of a highly contrasting color.

HALLWAYS AND STAIRWAYS

- In hallways, make sure that lighting is uniform throughout.
- Locate drinking fountains and fire extinguishers along only one wall throughout hallways to allow individuals who are visually impaired to trail the other wall without encountering obstacles.
- Install grab bars where they may be needed.
- Light stairwells clearly.
- Make certain that stairway railings extend beyond the top and bottom steps.
- Mark landings in a highly contrasting color.

SIGNS

- Place all signs at eye level, with large lettering according to specifications outlined in the Americans with Disabilities Act (ADA).
- Provide braille signage according to ADA specifications.
- Mark emergency exits clearly.
- When making signs by hand, use a heavy black felt-tip pen on a white, off-white, or light-yellow nonglossy background.

TELEPHONES

- Provide some telephones with large-print keypads.
- Provide telephone amplifiers that increase the level of sound.

These basic environmental design and safety tips can go a long way toward making your facility a comfortable and accessible environment for older persons who are visually impaired, and for everyone else who uses the facility and services.

MODIFICATIONS TO THE LIVING ENVIRONMENT

The environmental elements described here are also important for the older person with impaired vision to function independently and safely at home. Within the vision rehabilitation field, rehabilitation teachers, professionals who teach adaptive techniques for independent living, work with older persons who are visually impaired to make these environmental modifications within the living environment and in the workplace.

A rehabilitation teacher who provides independent living skills training in the older person's living environment can also assess the environment for safety and ease of functioning. Suggestions for modifications are usually easy to carry out because they typically involve no- or low-cost changes, which make modifications possible for older people with a range of personal incomes.

APPENDIX F

An Environmental Checklist

It is critical to make the rooms or apartments of older residents with visual impairments, as well as the public areas of the facility, safe and accessible. Lighting, color contrast, appropriate signage, and reduction of glare are important factors to consider.

You can use the following checklist to assess the environment of your facility for safety and accessibility. It is best to conduct this review of your facility with pen in hand. It would be a good idea for at least one staff person to tour the facility wearing a variety of vision simulators before completing the checklist. For example, the problems that glare can cause in seeing objects may not be as easy to spot without the simulators.

After conducting the review, use the lists in Appendix E and the tips in Appendix C for suggested solutions to any of the problems you may encounter. You may need to discuss needed changes with your supervisor.

A CHECKLIST FOR ENVIRONMENTAL SAFETY AND ACCESS

THE ENTRANCE

______ Are the curb and outside steps marked with a contrasting color?

______ Are glass doors marked to make them more visible?

______ If there is a revolving door, are there conventional doors on either side?

______ Does the wheelchair ramp have a nonslip surface?

PUBLIC TELEPHONE AREA

______ Is the area accessible from the most commonly used rooms?

______ Do telephone booths protrude into traffic areas?

______ Do some of the telephones have large-print dials?

______ Are telephone amplifiers, which increase the level of sound, available?

MAILBOX AREA

______ Is the area brightly lit?

______ Are the names and numbers easy to read?

______ Are the boxes that belong to residents who are visually impaired identified with a bright dot or a label?

HALLWAYS

______ Is lighting uniform throughout? Is there glare in any area?

______ Do doors contrast in color with walls; do the baseboards contrast in color with walls?

______ Are drinking fountains and fire extinguishers located along one wall only and recessed?

______ Is equipment lying around in the halls?

______ Are ramps identifiable by a tactile change in surface?

______ Are emergency exits clearly marked?

______ Are floors waxed with a nonglare, nonslippery wax?

______ Are signs at eye level? Is there adequate lighting to read them? Is the print large enough to be read?

STAIRWAYS AND ELEVATORS

______ Are stairways clearly lit?

______ Are landings marked in a contrasting color?

______ Are the Up and Down light indicators of elevators easy to see?

______ Can floor buttons in elevators be identified by both sight and touch?

______ Are floors also identified by an audible signal or are the floors announced?

RECREATION ROOMS, DINING ROOMS, AND OTHER COMMON ROOMS

______ Are there multiple sources of light throughout the room?

______ Is there natural light?

______ Do furniture, carpeting, and walls contrast with each other? Has textured carpeting been used that makes walking difficult?

______ Is there furniture in high-traffic areas?

______ Are dining room chairs pushed in under the tables?

______ Do windows have adjustable drapes, shades, or blinds to eliminate or reduce glare?

______ Are floors waxed with nonslippery, nonglare wax?

COMMON BATHROOMS

______ Are the signs identifying the men's room and the women's room large enough to read and easy to feel? Are they at eye level?

______ Do fixtures contrast in color with walls and floors?

______ Are there grab bars along the wall, on the bathtub, and in the shower?

______ Are the cold- and hot-water faucets clearly marked?

______ Are rugs and bath mats nonskid?

______ Has glare been reduced to a minimum?

______ Are there things that can be done to increase contrast?

THE RESIDENT'S LIVING QUARTERS

When reviewing a resident's living quarters, be sure to complete this checklist together with the resident to make sure that any changes meet the approval and vision requirements of the resident.

______ Is there adequate lighting for the resident to read, write, and carry out other tasks in the kitchen and bathroom?

______ Is glare a problem? What about from mirrors? Windows? Flooring?

______ Are rugs and bath mats nonskid?

______ Is the threshold flush with the floor?

______ Has color contrast been used effectively with walls, woodwork, floor coverings, and cabinet surfaces in the kitchen and bathroom?

______ Is the TV located in a place where the resident can see it—away from glare? Close enough to see? With appropriate lighting?

______ Is there furniture in the middle of the living room floor or bedroom floor?

APPENDIX G

Independent Living Services for Older Individuals Who Are Blind

This appendix provides a listing of programs in each state under the federal Independent Living Services for Older Individuals Who Are Blind legislation. These programs are designed to help older individuals who are blind or visually impaired, to enable them to continue living as independently as possible. Some of the core services include training for activities of daily living, provision of adaptive devices, training in the use of a white cane, training in communication skills, and provision of low vision services and devices. Eligibility for services and the specific services offered vary from state to state. Some states do not serve individuals in assisted living settings.

STATE REHABILITATION AGENCIES

To locate the Independent Living Services for Older Individuals Who Are Blind program in your state, contact your state rehabilitation agency and ask for the Chapter 2 Program Manager.

ALABAMA DEPARTMENT OF REHABILITATION SERVICES
2129 East South Boulevard
Montgomery, AL 36116-2455
Local Telephone: (334) 281-8780
Toll Free Telephone: (800) 441-7607
URL: http://www.rehab.state.al.us

ALASKA DEPARTMENT OF LABOR:
DIVISION OF VOCATIONAL REHABILITATION
801 West 10th Avenue, Suite A
Juneau, AK 99801
Local Telephone: (907) 465-2814
Toll Free Telephone: (800) 478-2815
URL: http://www.labor.state.ak.us/dvr/home.htm

ARIZONA DEPARTMENT OF ECONOMIC SECURITY:
REHABILITATION SERVICES ADMINISTRATION
1789 West Jefferson Street, 930A
Phoenix, AZ 85007
Local Telephone: (602) 542-6289
Toll Free Telephone: (800) 563-1221
TDD/TTY Telephone: (520)628-6864
URL: http://www.de.state.az.us

ARKANSAS DEPARTMENT OF HUMAN SERVICES:
DIVISION OF SERVICES FOR THE BLIND
522 Main Street, Suite 100
Little Rock, AR 72203-3237
Local Telephone: (501) 682-5463
Toll Free Telephone: (800) 960-9270
URL: http://www.state.ar.us/dhs/dsb

CALIFORNIA DEPARTMENT OF REHABILITATION:
SERVICES FOR THE BLIND
2000 Evergreen Street
Sacramento, CA 95815-3832
Local Telephone: (916) 263-8953
TDD/TTY Telephone: (530) 345-3897
URL: http://www.rehab.cahwnet.gov/

COLORADO DEPARTMENT OF HUMAN SERVICES:
REHABILITATION SERVICES
2211 West Evans Street, Building B
Denver, CO 80230
Local Telephone: (720) 884-1231
URL: http://www.state.co.us

CONNECTICUT STATE BOARD OF EDUCATION AND SERVICES FOR THE BLIND
184 Windsor Avenue
Windsor, CT 06095
Local Telephone: (860) 602-4000
Toll Free Telephone: (800) 842-4510
TDD/TTY Telephone: (860) 602-4002
URL: http://www.besb.state.ct.us/

DELAWARE DEPARTMENT OF HEALTH AND SOCIAL SERVICES:
DIVISION FOR THE VISUALLY IMPAIRED
1901 North DuPont Highway
Biggs Building
New Castle, DE 19720
Local Telephone: (302) 577-4730
TDD/TTY Telephone: (302) 577-4750
URL: http://www.state.de.us/dhss/dvi/dvihome.htm

DISTRICT OF COLUMBIA DEPARTMENT OF HUMAN SERVICES:
REHABILITATION SERVICES ADMINISTRATION
810 First Street, NE, 10th Floor
Washington, DC 20002
Local Telephone: (202) 442-8663
URL: http://www.dhs.washington.dc.us

FLORIDA DEPARTMENT OF EDUCATION:
DIVISION OF BLIND SERVICES
2551 Executive Center Circle
Tallahassee, FL 32399
Local Telephone: (850) 488-1330
Toll Free Telephone: (800) 342-1828
URL: http://www.state.fl.us/dbs

GEORGIA DEPARTMENT OF LABOR:
DIVISION OF REHABILITATION SERVICES
Two Peachtree Stree NW
Suite 35-412
Atlanta, GA 30303-3142
Local Telephone: (404) 657-3000
URL: http://www.vocrehabga.org

HAWAII DEPARTMENT OF HUMAN SERVICES:
HO'OPONO SERVICES FOR THE BLIND, VOCATIONAL REHABILITATION AND SERVICES FOR THE BLIND DIVISION
1901 Bachelor Street
Honolulu, HI 96817
Local Telephone: (808) 692-7716
URL: http://www.rrhi.com/hooponoblindservices

IDAHO COMMISSION FOR THE BLIND AND VISUALLY IMPAIRED
341 West Washington Street
Boise, ID 83702-0012
Local Telephone: (208) 334-3220
URL: http://www.icbvi.state.id.us

ILLINOIS DEPARTMENT OF REHABILITATION SERVICES:
BUREAU OF BLIND SERVICES
623 East Adams Street
Springfield, IL 62794-9429
Local Telephone: (217) 785-3887
Toll Free Telephone: (800) 275-3677
TTD/TTY Telephone: (630) 495-2294
URL: http://www.state.il.us/agency/dhs/bsnp.html

INDIANA FAMILY AND SOCIAL SERVICES ADMINISTRATION:
DIVISION OF DISABILITY, AGING AND REHABILITATIVE SERVICES
Indiana Government Center
402 West Washington Street
Room W-453
Indianapolis, IN 46204
Local Telephone: (317) 232-7020
Toll Free Telephone: (800) 545-7763
URL: http://www.state.in.us/fssa/

IOWA DEPARTMENT FOR THE BLIND
524 Fourth Street
Des Moines, IA 50309-2364
Local Telephone: (515) 281-1333
Toll Free Telephone: (800) 362-2587
TDD/TTY Telephone: (515) 281-1355
URL: http://www.blind.state.ia.us/

KANSAS DEPARTMENT OF SOCIAL AND REHABILITATION SERVICES:
DIVISION OF SERVICES FOR THE BLIND, REHABILITATION CENTER FOR THE BLIND
2516 SW Sixth Avenue
Topeka, KS 66606
Local Telephone: (785) 296-3311
URL: http://www.state.ks.us/public/srs/

KENTUCKY DEPARTMENT FOR THE BLIND
209 St. Clair Street
Frankfort, KY 40601
Local Telephone: (502) 564-4754
Toll Free Telephone: (800) 334-6920
URL: http://www.state.ky.us/agencies/wforce/dfbliind/index.htm

LOUISIANA DEPARTMENT OF SOCIAL SERVICES:
LOUISIANA REHABILITATION SERVICES
8225 Florida Boulevard
Baton Rouge, LA 70806
Local Telephone: (225) 925-3594
Toll Free Telephone: (800) 737-2958
URL: http://www.dss.state.la.us/offlrs/

MAINE DEPARTMENT OF LABOR:
DIVISION FOR THE BLIND AND VISUALLY IMPAIRED
2 Anthony Avenue
#150 State House Station
Augusta, ME 04333-0150
Local Telephone: (207) 624-5959
TDD/TTY Telephone: (207) 624-5955
URL: http://www.state.me.us/rehab/

MARYLAND STATE DEPARTMENT OF EDUCATION:
DIVISION OF REHABILITATION SERVICES
2301 Argonne Drive
Baltimore, MD 21218-1696
Local Telephone: (410) 554-9405
Toll Free Telephone: (888) 220-7117
TDD/TTY Telephone: (410) 554-9411
URL: http://www.dors.state.md.us/

MASSACHUSETTS STATE COMMISSION FOR THE BLIND
88 Kingston Street
Boston, MA 02111-2227
Local Telephone: (617) 727-5550
Toll Free Telephone: (800) 392-6450
URL: http://www.magnet.state.ma.us/mcb

MICHIGAN COMMISSION FOR THE BLIND:
FAMILY INDEPENDENCE AGENCY
201 North Washington Square
Lansing, MI 48933
Local Telephone: (313) 256-1524
Toll Free Telephone: (800) 292-4200
URL: http://www.mfia.state.us/

MINNESOTA STATE SERVICES FOR THE BLIND
2200 University Avenue West
Suite 240
St. Paul, MN 55114-1840
Local Telephone: (651) 642-0838
Toll Free Telephone: (800) 652-9000
TTD/TTY Telephone: (651) 642-0506
URL: http://www.mnworkforcecenter. org/ssb/

MISSISSIPPI DEPARTMENT OF REHABILITATION SERVICES:
OFFICE OF VOCATIONAL REHABILITATION FOR THE BLIND
1281 Highway 51 North
Madison, MS 39110
Local Telephone: (601) 853-5245
Toll Free Telephone: (800) 443-1000
URL: http://www.mdrs.state.ms.us

MISSOURI REHABILITATION SERVICES FOR THE BLIND
3418 Knipp Drive
Jefferson City, MO 65109
Local Telephone: (573) 751-4249
Toll Free Telephone: (800) 592-6004
URL: http://www.dss.state.mo.us/dfs/rehab.htm

MONTANA DEPARTMENT OF PUBLIC HEALTH AND HUMAN SERVICES:
DEVELOPMENTAL DISABLITIES PROGRAM/ VOCATIONAL REHABILITATION/ BLIND AND LOW VISION SERVICES
111 North Sanders, Room 307
Helena, MT 59604
Local Telephone: (406) 444-2590
Toll Free Telephone: (877) 296-1197

NEBRASKA COMMISSION FOR THE BLIND AND VISUALLY IMPAIRED
4600 Valley Road
Suite 100
Lincoln, NE 68510-4840
Local Telephone: (402) 471-8105
Toll Free Telephone: (877) 809-2419
TTD/TTY Telephone: (402) 471-2891
URL: http://www.ncbvi.state.ne.us/

NEVADA BUREAU OF SERVICES TO THE BLIND AND VISUALLY IMPAIRED
505 East King Street, Room 505
Carson City, NV 89701
Local Telephone: (775)684-4244
Toll Free Telephone: (800) 607-6564
TDD/TTY Telephone: (800) 684-8626
URL: http://www.detr.state.nv.us/rehab/reh_bvi.htm

NEW HAMPSHIRE DIVISION OF VOCATIONAL REHABILITATION:
SERVICES FOR THE BLIND AND VISUALLY IMPAIRED
78 Regional Drive
Building 2
Concord, NH 03301
Local Telephone: (603) 271-3537
Toll Free Telephone: (800) 581-6881
URL: http://216.64.49.52/vrweb/blind.html

NEW JERSEY COMMISSION FOR THE BLIND AND VISUALLY IMPAIRED
153 Halsey Street, 6th Floor
Newark, NJ 07101
Local Telephone: (973) 648-3333

NEW MEXICO COMMISSION FOR THE BLIND
1120 Paseo de Peralta
PERA Building, Room 553
Santa Fe, NM 87504
Local Telephone: (505) 827-4479
Toll Free Telephone: (888) 513-7968
URL: http://www.state.nm.us/cftb

NEW YORK STATE OFFICE OF CHILDREN AND FAMILY SERVICES:
COMMISSION FOR THE BLIND AND VISUALLY HANDICAPPED
40 North Pearl Street
Albany, NY 12243
Local Telephone: (518) 474-6812
TDD/TTY Telephone: (518) 474-7501
URL: http://www.dfa.state.ny.us/cbvh

NORTH CAROLINA DIVISION OF SERVICES FOR THE BLIND
2601 Mail Service Center
309 Ashe Avenue
Raleigh, NC 27699-2601
Local Telephone: (919) 733-9822
TDD/TTY Telephone: (919) 733-9700
URL: http://www.dhhs.state.nc.us/dsb/

OHIO REHABILITATION SERVICES COMMISSION:
BUREAU OF SERVICES FOR THE VISUALLY IMPAIRED
400 East Campus View Boulevard
Columbus, OH 43235-4604
Local Telephone: (614) 438-1255
Toll Free Telephone: (800) 282-4536
TDD/TTY Telephone: (614) 995-1161
URL: http://www.state.oh.us/rsc

OKLAHOMA DEPARTMENT OF REHABILITATION SERVICES
3535 NW 58th Street
Suite 500
Oklahoma City, OK 73112
Local Telephone: (405) 951-3400
Toll Free Telephone: (800) 845-8476
URL: http://www.onenet.net/~drspiowm

OREGON COMMISSION FOR THE BLIND
535 12th Avenue SE
Portland, OR 97214
Local Telephone: (503) 731-3221
Toll Free Telephone: (888) 202-5463
TDD/TTY Telephone: (503) 731-3224
URL: http://www.cfb.state.or.us

PUERTO RICO DEPARTMENT OF LABOR:
VOCATIONAL REHABILITIATION ADMINISTRATION
PO Box 191118
San Juan, PR 00919-1118
Local Telephone: (787) 729-0160

RHODE ISLAND DEPARTMENT OF HUMAN SERVICES:
SERVICES FOR THE BLIND AND VISUALLY IMPAIRED
40 Fountain Street
Providence, RI 02903-1898
Local Telephone: (401) 277-2382
Toll Free Telephone: (800) 752-8088
URL: http://www.ors.state.ri.us

SOUTH CAROLINA COMMISSION FOR THE BLIND
P.O. Box 79
Columbia, SC 29202-0079
Local Telephone: (803) 898-8700
Toll Free Telephone: (800) 922-2222
URL: http://www.sccb.state.sc.us

SOUTH DAKOTA DEPARTMENT OF HUMAN SERVICES:
DIVISION OF SERVICE TO THE BLIND AND VISUALLY IMPAIRED
3800 East Highway 34
500 East Capitol
Pierre, SD 57501-5070
Local Telephone: (605) 773-4644
Toll Free Telephone: (800) 265-9684
URL: http://www.state.sd.us/dhs/

TENNESSEE SERVICES FOR THE BLIND AND VISUALLY IMPAIRED
400 Deaderick Street
11th Flooor
Nashville, TN 37248-6200
Local Telephone: (615) 313-4914

TEXAS COMMISSION FOR THE BLIND
4800 North Lamar Boulevard
Austin, TX 78756-3178
Local Telephone: (512) 377-0500
Toll Free Telephone: (800) 252-5204
TDD/TTY Telephone: (512) 377-0546
URL: http://www.tcb.state.tx.us/

UTAH DIVISION OF SERVICES FOR THE BLIND AND VISUALLY IMPAIRED
250 North 1950 West, Suite B
Salt Lake City, UT 84116-7902
Local Telephone: (801) 323-4343
Toll Free Telephone: (800) 284-1823
TDD/TTY Telephone: (801) 323-4395

VERMONT AGENCY OF HUMAN SERVICES:
DIVISION FOR THE BLIND AND VISUALLY IMPAIRED
Osgood Building
103 South Maine Street
Waterbury, VT 05671
Local Telephone: (802) 241-2210
URL: http://www.dad.state.vt.us/dbvi

VIRGIN ISLANDS DEPARTMENT OF HUMAN SERVICES
Knud Hansen Complex
Building A-1303
Hospital Ground
St. Thomas, VI 00802
Local Telephone: (340) 774-0930
URL: http://www.usvi.org/humanservices/index.html

VIRGINIA DEPARTMENT FOR THE BLIND AND VISION IMPAIRED
397 Azalea Avenue
Richmond, VA 23227-3623
Local Telephone: (804) 371-3140
URL: http://www.vdbvi.org

WASHINGTON STATE DEPARTMENT OF SERVICES FOR THE BLIND
402 Legion Way, SE
Suite 100
Olympia, WA 98504-0933
Local Telephone: (360) 586-1224
Toll Free Telephone: (800) 552-7103
TDD/TTY Telephone: (206) 764-4051
URL: http://www.wa.gov/dsb

WEST VIRGINIA DEPARTMENT OF EDUCATION AND THE ARTS:
DIVISION OF REHABILITATION SERVICES, INFORMATION AND REFERRAL SERVICES FOR THE BLIND AND VISUALLY IMPAIRED
P.O. Box 50890
State Capitol Complex
Charleston, WV 25305-0890
Local Telephone: (304) 766-4891
Toll Free Telephone: (800) 642-3021
TDD/TTY Telephone: (304) 766-4970

WISCONSIN DEPARTMENT OF WORKFORCE DEVELOPMENT:
DIVISION OF VOCATIONAL REHABILITATION
2917 International Lane
Suite 300
Madison, WI 53707-7852
Local Telephone: (608) 243-5600
Toll Free Telephone: (800) 442-3477
TDD/TTY Telephone: (608) 243-5601
URL: http://www.dwd.state.wi.us/dvr

WYOMING DIVISION OF VOCATIONAL REHABILITATION
1100 Herschler Building
Cheyenne, WY 82002
Local Telephone: (307) 777-7389
URL: http://www.onestop.state.wy.us/appview/ujn-home.asp

About the Authors

ALBERTA L. ORR, M.S.W., C.S.W., is the director of the National Aging Program of the American Foundation for the Blind (AFB) in New York City and convener of the National Aging and Vision Network, spearheading the National Agenda on Vision and Aging. She is also an adjunct faculty member at Hunter College of the City University of New York, where she teaches in the Rehabilitation Teaching master's degree program, Department of Special Education. She has served as the principal investigator for many federally funded projects and is the author of numerous publications, including *Vision and Aging: Crossroads for Service Delivery* and *Issues in Aging and Vision: A Curriculum for University Programs and In-Service Training*, and has produced several videos, including *Profiles in Aging and Vision*.

PRISCILLA ROGERS, Ph.D., is currently a consultant to the National Aging Program of the American Foundation for the Blind. She is the former commissioner of blind services in Kentucky and held the position of bureau chief of client services in Florida, including programs for older persons with visual impairments. Her master's degree is in gerontology and her doctorate is in special education with a specialization in visual impairment and aging. She has authored several articles on vision and aging and co-authored several curricula. She has served as chief investigator on several federal grants.

Index

Index

Index